THE·BUSINESS·SIDE·OF·GENERAL·PRACTICE

Making Sense of Partnerships

EDITED BY
NORMAN ELLIS and TONY STANTON

Foreword by
IAN BOGLE
Chairman, General Medical Services Committee,
British Medical Association

RADCLIFFE MEDICAL PRESS
OXFORD and NEW YORK

© 1994 Radcliffe Medical Press Ltd
15 Kings Meadow, Ferry Hinksey Road, Oxford OX2 0DP

Radcliffe Medical Press Inc
141 Fifth Avenue, Suite N, NY 10010, USA

All rights reserved. No part of this publication may be reproduced, stored in a retrieval system, or transmitted in any form or by any means, electronic, mechanical, photocopying, recording or otherwise without the prior permission of the copyright owner.

A catalogue record for this book is available from the British Library.

ISBN 1 870905 62 8

Typeset by Advance Typesetting Ltd, Oxford
Printed and bound in Great Britain by Biddles Ltd, Guildford & King's Lynn

Contents

	Foreword	v
	List of Contributors	vii
	The Business Side of General Practice: Editorial Board	ix
	Preface	xi
1.	Why work in a partnership?	1
2.	The partnership agreement	7
3.	When partners fall out: legal remedies	27
4.	Is your partnership working? The role of mediation	35
5.	Partnership accounts	43
6.	Partnership taxation	63
7.	Exploitation in partnerships	81
8.	Sharing workload and profits	93
9.	Improving partnership agreements	101
10.	Future developments	109
	Index	115

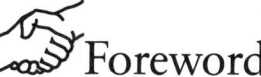Foreword

A large and increasing majority of GPs work in partnerships. This legal, professional and financial relationship is a major feature of most of our working lives. It is also the feature of general practice that is most prone to becoming a major source of conflict and dispute. Indeed, during my 19 years' experience as an LMC secretary, the most acrimonious disputes were almost invariably between partners, sometimes leading to costly (and often pointless) litigation which usually failed to resolve anything and left all parties equally disgruntled.

Partnerships disputes can be avoided. This book contains valuable advice and information on how we can improve on the working arrangements within partnerships. It brings together the experience of both professional advisers and GPs themselves. Each chapter offers valuable insights into partnership problems. It does not (and indeed should not) offer a single remedy or solution; such a panacea does not exist, and practitioners and partnerships have to work out for themselves what arrangements best suit their circumstances. However, when tackling this important task, this book is essential reading and a useful source document.

IAN BOGLE
Chairman
General Medical Services Committee
British Medical Association

Making Sense of Partnerships

Contributors

LYNNE ABBESS, *Solicitor, Hempsons*

LORNA DUNLOP, *General Practitioner; Member, Scottish General Medical Services Committee, British Medical Association*

NORMAN ELLIS, *Under Secretary, British Medical Association*

SIMON FRADD, *General Practitioner; Member of Negotiating Team and Chairman of Partnership Agreements Working Group, General Medical Services Committee, British Medical Association; former Member, Medical Practices Committee*

NICK GILD, *Solicitor; Senior Lecturer, Thames Valley University, London*

CHRIS HUGHES, *Solicitor; Head of Legal Services, British Medical Association*

VALERIE MARTIN, *Accountant, Pannell Kerr Forster*

TONY STANTON, *Secretary, London Local Medical Committees; former Deputy Chairman, General Medical Services Committee, British Medical Association*

The Business Side of General Practice

Editorial Board for Making Sense of Partnerships

STUART CARNE, *former President, Royal College of General Practitioners*

HEATHER NORGOVE, *Association of Health Centre and Practice Administrators*

Editorial Board for the Series

STUART CARNE, *former President, Royal College of General Practitioners*

JOHN CHISHOLM, *Joint Deputy Chairman and Negotiator, General Medical Services Committee, British Medical Association*

NORMAN ELLIS, *Under Secretary, British Medical Association*

EILEEN FARRANT, *former Chairman, Association of Medical Secretaries, Practice Administrators and Receptionists*

WILLIAM KENT, *Secretary, General Medical Services Committee, British Medical Association*

CLIVE PARR, *General Manager, Hereford and Worcester Family Health Services Authority*

DAVID TAYLOR, *Head of Health Care Quality, Audit Commission*

CHARLES ZUCKERMAN, *Secretary, Birmingham Local Medical Committee; Member, General Medical Services Committee, British Medical Association*

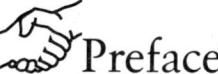Preface

THE joint editors believe this book fills an important gap in the range of publications on the Business Side of General Practice. Indeed, it is surprising that there is not already a comparable text devoted solely to the subject of GP partnerships, bearing in mind that they are such a major source of conflict and disputes. Of course, there have been numerous articles in the medico-political press (many of which have been written by the authors of this book) dealing with various specific aspects of partnerships. The particular value of this book is that it brings together between one set of covers a group of authors who together have an extensive body of knowledge and experience on partnership matters.

The book's aims are both 'preventive' and 'curative' – to use a heavily overworked clinical analogy. It is 'preventive' in that it offers advice, which if followed should avoid many of the pitfalls and problems of partnerships; obvious examples are the detailed descriptions of what should be included in a written partnership deed, and how to organize a partnership's accounts and taxation. Its 'curative' role is evident in those chapters which discuss how to improve partnership agreements and various ways of resolving partnership disputes.

It is both unsurprising and reassuring that the same basic facts and messages are reiterated throughout the book, although each author puts his or her slant on them. All of the authors stress that partnerships should:

- be based on equitable working relationships
- have a comprehensive written agreement
- follow sound accounting procedures and make adequate provision for their tax liabilities
- ensure that good communications between the partners are maintained, for example by means of regular partnership meetings.

Finally, where should an individual doctor or a partnership turn for advice and assistance? These can be obtained from many expert sources, including BMA regional offices, local medical committee secretaries, accountants and solicitors.

NORMAN ELLIS
TONY STANTON
January 1994

1 Why Work in a Partnership?

Tony Stanton

GENERAL practice is recognized as a high stress occupation and one factor which can contribute to this is being a member of a partnership. Most partnerships work tolerably well; some operate as tightly knit teams; many are generally unhappy, but nevertheless struggle on. A few partnerships are disaster areas, descending through a spiral of backbiting and arguments to letters from lawyers, finally ending in legal action often with calamitous financial consequences.

Despite all these reservations, most general practitioners work in partnerships; the proportion who do so continues to increase and the size of the partnerships themselves is also rising.

By 1990, some 33 000 doctors were working in NHS general practice in Britain, a figure which includes all types of GP – principals, assistants and trainees. Over 30 000 of these were unrestricted principals, providing the full range of general medical services.

During the period 1970–90, when the old GP contract still applied, an increasing proportion of doctors worked in partnerships and the average size of these rose substantially. In 1970, 21% of GPs were single-handed, a proportion which had fallen to 11.5% by 1990. During the same period, the percentage of GPs working in partnerships of four or more rose from 28% to 55%. Even more dramatically, the proportion of GPs in partnerships of six or more increased from 5% in 1970 to over 21% in 1990. Figure 1 clearly illustrates the overall trends: a halving of the proportion of single-handed doctors, a steady decline in partnerships of three or fewer, and a marked growth in partnerships of four or more.

Why have these changes occurred? There are several obvious explanations. First the structure and funding of NHS general practice has led to the overwhelming majority of GPs becoming principals. Having completed their vocational training, those doctors intending to become NHS GPs have to choose between working for an employer (usually another GP) as a salaried employee or becoming a principal on the medical list of an FHSA

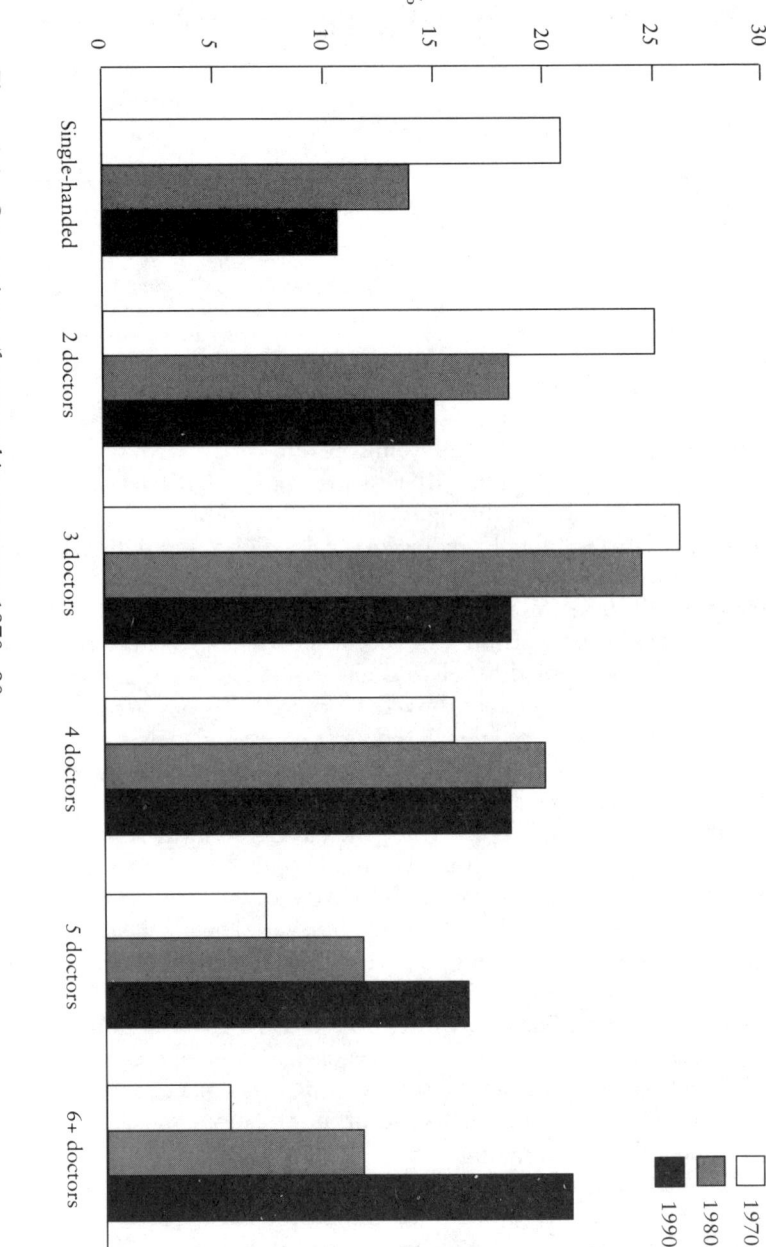

Figure 1.1 Comparison of partnership structures 1970–90

or Health Board. There are two main ways in which a doctor can be admitted to an FHSA/Health Board medical list; either by becoming a single-handed doctor or by joining an existing partnership.

It is far from easy to become a single-handed practitioner; the only three ways of doing it are by:

- applying for an advertised vacancy
- breaking away from an existing partnership
- establishing an entirely new practice.

Seeking to become a single-handed practitioner other than by succeeding to an existing list is fraught with difficulties. Breaking away from an existing partnership has several practical obstacles, including the often insurmountable problems of obtaining suitable premises, the increasing constraints imposed by cash limits on practice staff, and escaping from the terms of any restrictive covenant.

Contrary to popular belief, restrictive covenants are enforceable in NHS general practice. In one sense, the only asset common to all practices is the goodwill embodied in the patient list. The NHS Act prohibits the sale or purchase of this goodwill, but not its existence.

Establishing an entirely new single-handed practice is subject not only to the usual commercial risks but to NHS manpower controls exercised by the Medical Practices Committee (MPC). Before the MPC was established in 1948 by the NHS Act, the more desirable parts of England and Wales had more than enough family doctors. Elsewhere, by contrast, some 50% of the population lived in severely under-doctored areas where average list sizes exceeded 3500 per GP, sometimes by more than a factor of two.

The MPC does not have the power to direct doctors to a particular area, but it can tell them where they may not practise. As a consequence, a doctor wishing to start a new single-handed practice may normally do so only in an area designated by the MPC as being 'open', ie less than adequately doctored. Paradoxically, because the MPC has been so successful in achieving an even spread of GPs across England and Wales, the proportion of these countries currently designated as 'open' is at an all time low. (There is a separate MPC for Scotland, and Northern Ireland has its own similar arrangements.)

Although by definition 'open' areas are relatively under-doctored, there is no guarantee that a new practitioner will be able to establish a viable practice. Difficulties in finding premises, raising finance and obtaining adequate reimbursement of expenses are major obstacles that need to be overcome.

Thus the decline in the number of single-handed doctors has become a self-perpetuating trend. The development strategies of FHSAs, even when the local medical committees and community health councils are taken into account, mean that this trend is likely to continue to accelerate.

Therefore, most doctors entering general practice as a career have little choice other than to join an existing partnership. This solves many problems for the individual doctor. It provides a sound economic basis for practice at an early stage in the career, ie a share of the income of an established practice derived largely from the capitation payments received from the FHSA, which in turn reflect the number of patients on its list. It also provides premises from which to work. As has been pointed out, the difficulties in obtaining surgery accommodation probably constitute the single biggest hurdle facing a new GP; even if a list of patients and the ensuing NHS income are both assured, premises are rarely easy to find. Doctors retiring from single-handed practice often have surgeries which are either part of their residence or leased from a landlord; in neither case are they normally available to a succeeding doctor.

A third major attraction of joining an existing practice is the professional support it offers; it involves close working relations with doctor colleagues and ensures that the GP's clinical work is complemented by a primary health care team.

The 1990 GP contract has added to the complexities of general practice. It was devised to make patient list size a more effective determinant of a doctor's income by accentuating both capitation payments and bonus payments based on practice populations. Successive changes in the Statement of Fees and Allowances (SFA) reflect this trend. The paradox of this growing trend towards partnerships is that within neither the NHS Regulations nor the SFA is much said about partnerships as such. Indeed, most of what is said is essentially negative, being more helpful for defining when a doctor is *not* a partner.

The whole area of partnership in NHS general practice needs to be reviewed. As with all types of partnership, it is subject to the provisions of the Partnership Act 1890. In addition, it is an association between professional medical colleagues. Finally, it has become inextricably linked with the NHS payment system.

It is this last point which has led to the raison d'être of this book. Most GPs join an existing partnership as a partner from the outset. This is different to the procedure in other established professions. For example, solicitors and accountants tend to join their respective firms as salaried employees and only achieve partnership status after several years.

The organization of NHS general practice and its payment system, in particular the basic practice allowance and its associated allowances, have encouraged this trend. While no-one wishes to see a return to the days of 'assistants without a view', the interest shown in developing practice based contracts suggests that there is a case for arguing that allowing individual freedom under the umbrella of shared costs and shared support might make for happier GPs and happier patients.

2 The Partnership Agreement

Norman Ellis

THE partnership provides a legal framework within which most GPs work: less than 10% of practices are single-handed. Given its importance to the business of general practice, it is remarkable how widespread ignorance and neglect of the partnership agreement is in the profession.

Many practices do not have written partnership agreements; it has been estimated that at least half either have no written agreement or work to an outdated model. Any partnership without this essential documentation is susceptible to the vagaries that flow from the fact that relations between partners are strictly controlled by a century-old statute, the Partnership Act 1890. A partnership without a written agreement is known as a 'partnership at will' and is governed by this Act. Its main characteristics are listed in Box 2.1.

A partnership can develop the rules drawn from this legislation or agree to abide by additional rules too. Variations and departures from the Partnership Act can be inferred from the conduct of the partners; for example, although the Act requires profits to be shared equally, many practices opt for a different basis of division.

Given the dangers and potential difficulties of a 'partnership at will', it is surprising that so many practices do not have written agreements. However, neglect of essential paperwork is not uncommon in general practice. Until comparatively recently a large majority of practice staff did not have written employment contracts, even though they were legally entitled to them.

The need for a written agreement

A partnership in any field of activity can be plagued by problems, and general practice is no exception. Although a written agreement offers no panacea, it at least lays down ground rules which can help to resolve, if not

> **Box 2.1: Key characteristics of a 'partnership at will'**
>
> - The entire partnership automatically ends upon the death, retirement or bankruptcy of any one partner.
> - Any partner can choose to end the partnership immediately without notice to the other partners, unless remaining partners elect to continue.
> - The partners must share profits (and losses) equally.
> - All partners must have free access to the bank account and are entitled to take part in managing the business.
> - Partnership decisions may be made by a majority of the partners, except that all partners must consent to a new partner being admitted as well as any change in the nature of the business.
> - No partner can be expelled from the partnership.
> - Partners must not compete with the partnership; if they engage in any business on their own account in the same broad field of activity as the partnership, any income from this must be paid to the partnership.
> - All partners are regarded as 'agents' of the partnership and can take decisions and enter into commitments to which the partnership is bound (eg ordering computer equipment).
> - All partners are liable for everything for which the partnership is liable and for the acts of individual partners carried out in the course of the partnership.

avoid, problems. Once these rules are established, it is only sensible to take it a step further by writing them down clearly and unambiguously so that all partners know exactly where they stand.

Partnership disputes are widespread and can present intractable problems. GP partnerships typically experience such problems and difficulties, and the imposition of the 1990 contract has added greatly to these by imposing extra pressures on the practice and many partnerships have been tested to destruction by its exigencies. Whilst an agreement cannot prevent disputes from occurring, it can help to avoid many common problems and can frequently resolve those which occur by specifying the procedures to be followed when a dispute arises or a partnership breaks up.

What should be included in a written agreement?

A written agreement should not slavishly follow a prescribed standard format. It is vital that it reflects the wishes of the partners because only they know how they want to work together, the practice's circumstances and what problems need to be addressed.

No written agreement, no matter how comprehensive, can be expected to define all the rights and obligations of the partners; many of these have to be inferred from their day to day working relations. Nevertheless, there is a well-established framework that is widely used and this normally includes the clauses covered by the headings listed in Box 2.2. Strictly speaking, many of those standard clauses are not necessary because the rights or obligations they assign are either prescribed by the Partnership Act 1890, or they are always implied, for example the obligation to be just and faithful in all dealings with one's partners (*see* Figure 2.1). Nevertheless, it is usually advisable to include them in the agreement.

> 'A breach of good faith'
>
> A new partner joins a practice with a satisfactory partnership agreement. After two or three months, he suggests to the senior partner that it would be a good idea to employ a further practice nurse, adding that he knows someone who would be suitable. The senior partner agrees and the practice nurse is taken on. The nurse becomes pregnant and it is subsequently revealed that she is the live-in girlfriend of the new partner. In the opinion of the senior partner, a lot of patients are outraged by the situation, and he insists that the nurse stops work; in fact he wants to dismiss her. According to the partnership agreement, no member of staff can be dismissed without the agreement of all the partners, and therefore the nurse remains on the payroll until such time as she goes on maternity leave. The other partners override the junior partner's opposition on the grounds that his original action, in recommending his girlfriend as an employee without disclosing his relationship with her, was in breach of the obligation to act in good faith towards his partners.

Figure 2.1 A case study from the BMA files

> **Box 2.2: Main headings in a partnership agreement**
> - Date of document.
> - Name, title and address of the partnership.
> - Date of partnership commencement.
> - Nature of the practice's business.
> - Duration of partnership.
> - Practice premises.
> - Partnership capital.
> - Partnership expenses.
> - Partnership income.
> - Sharing the profits.
> - Attending to the affairs of the practice.
> - Management of practice staff.
> - Partnership decisions.
> - Partnership taxation.
> - Holidays and study leave.
> - Maternity provisions.
> - Prolonged incapacity and sickness.
> - Voluntary and compulsory retirement from the partnership.
> - Restrictive covenants.
> - Defence body membership.
> - Banking arrangements.
> - Accounts.
> - Arbitration/conciliation.

Date, name, title and address

Any agreement should specify a date of commencement which may precede the agreement if the partnership already exists, or be a future date if it is a new partnership. The agreement must be signed by all partners before it is dated. Any liability under the agreement will flow from the commencement date, not the date of agreement, unless the two are the same.

The agreement must also included the name under which the partnership will practise, and the address of the surgery premises. If the partnership uses any name which does not consist of the true surnames of all the partners, the true names of each partner must be included on letter headings, invoices, etc and displayed in each surgery, to meet the requirements of the Business Names Act 1985.

The nature of the business

A possible wording of this clause might be that the partners 'will carry on the profession of general medical practitioners'. It is essential to specify the nature of the business because this limits the extent to which each partner is liable as an agent of the firm. Otherwise, the liabilities arising from some other quite separate business activity undertaken by one partner might be incurred by all of the partners, even though they were not concerned in this other business.

> Extent of a partnership's liabilities
>
> A GP of 15 years standing, who had previously worked solely in a three-partner practice, started a business outside the practice with which the other two partners had no dealings financial or otherwise. In 1991, two years after the business started, it went into receivership.
>
> The GP's assets were liquidated to satisfy his personal debts, and these included his share in the partnership business, its equipment and premises, etc.
>
> Figure 2.2   A case study from the BMA files

Duration of the partnership

There is no advantage in limiting a partnership's duration; to do so reduces the security of all partners and could encourage them to compete among themselves in anticipation of the agreement's termination. Thus a partnership should be of indefinite duration: for the joint lives of all the partners or any two or more of them. Once a partnership is created, it can be dissolved at any time by mutual consent.

Practice premises

An incoming partner should clarify the ownership of any surgery premises and any prospective liability for the purchase of a share. If the existing partners have a large investment in the property and are seeking a

> **Box 2.3: Duration of a partnership**
>
> The Partnership Act 1890 states that every partnership is dissolved in respect of all the partners by the death or bankruptcy of any partner, unless there is an agreement to the contrary. This is why every partnership agreement covering more than two partners should include a provision to the contrary:
>
> > 'The partnership shall continue during the joint lives of the partners. The death, retirement, expulsion or bankruptcy of any partner shall not determine the partnership as regards the other partners.'

contribution from the new partner, then he or she should seek independent advice about funding from an accountant, a lawyer, or both.

A new partner who is buying an equal share of the premises is entitled to an equal share of FHSA or Health Board direct reimbursement under the rent and rates scheme, even though parity in profit share may not be reached for several years. This important matter is often neglected if a practice treats this reimbursement as normal income and pays it into the partnership account before calculating profit shares.

> **Box 2.4: Valuing the premises**
>
> A practice agreement should specify the basis on which the premises will be valued if a partner dies or resigns. Whatever basis is used, the agreement should state that goodwill must be excluded from the valuation.

The agreement should specify which partners are 'property owners'. If there is a lease or licence arrangement between the property owning partners and the other partners, it should be made only on the basis of legal advice. It is preferable that the agreement simply contains a provision defining the owners and confirming the rights of the others to use the practice premises, and that they should have a continuing right for, say, three months if the property owner(s) leave the partnership.

Rent and rates payments from the FHSA or Health Board should be paid into the partnership's bank account, being the property of the partnership as a whole.

Partnership capital/assets

This normally includes all property, equipment, drugs, surgery fittings and furniture, together with any cash used as working capital. An incoming partner will buy a share in these assets and also contribute to the practice's working capital. Partners normally own shares of the assets (apart from the premises) in the same proportion as their shares in the profits. The written agreement should specify how shares in partnership capital are divided among the partners and what constitutes the capital, and it should confirm the arrangements for expanding the capital.

> 'Acrimony over who owned what'
>
> Dr A fell out with his partners Drs B and C, and as a consequence dissolution of the partnership was discussed. There had been considerable discontent between the partners which arose from a long period of study leave taken by Dr A. The partnership did not have a written agreement. When discussions took place about the partnership break-up, it was extremely difficult to disentangle the capital of the partnership from items individually owned by the partners. This sadly led to the dispiriting scene of Dr A arguing in public with Drs B and C over who owned items of surgery equipment and furniture.
>
> There was no statement of the capital assets and no inventory which the three partners could use in their discussions about dissolution. Consequently, the process was accompanied by a lot of acrimony.

Figure 2.3   A case study from the BMA files

Partnership expenses

The agreement should also specify which expenses should be paid by the partnership as a whole. These should typically include the cost of practice staff, accounting and banking services, telephone and stationery, and the costs of occupying and running the premises (rent, rates, heating, lighting, cleaning and maintenance). All these shared expenses should be met before profits are calculated and distributed, and the partners should contribute to them in proportion to their profit shares. Other expenses, such as the costs of the partners' cars and house telephones, are normally paid by individual partners because this arrangement is usually fairer.

Whichever arrangement prevails, it should be clearly specified in the agreement; there should be no ambiguity or uncertainty about such crucial matters.

Partnership income

It is usually advisable to include all earnings from professional practice in the partnership income, otherwise individual partners might be encouraged to concentrate on those activities rewarded by personal rather than practice income and even compete among themselves for this type of work. However, certain earnings are often retained personally if these do not put at risk the collective efforts of the partnership, eg the seniority and postgraduate education allowances. Whatever arrangement is agreed, it must be equitable and should be defined in the partnership agreement.

It should nevertheless be emphasized that this is a traditional view of partnership income. Some partnerships have agreed equitable and amicable arrangements which allow individual partners to retain personally any income earned outside NHS general practice. This approach to defining partnership earnings may be particularly appropriate in partnerships where one or more partners have a less than full-time commitment.

> 'A learning experience'
>
> A new partner unwittingly signed a partnership agreement which allowed the other two partners to retain their seniority allowances and PGEAs, but required her PGEA to be paid into the 'pool' for distribution among all partners.

Figure 2.4 A case study from the BMA files

It is important that if a particular source of income (eg PGEA or hospital session payment) is retained by one partner, all other partners should enjoy the same right to retain earnings from the same or comparable sources of income.

Dividing the profits

Stated simply, the profit or loss is the difference between practice income and practice expenses. The agreement should specify the size of each partner's share of the profits, any future changes in the share, and the method of calculation and payment.

Under NHS regulations, for the FHSA or Health Board to recognize a GP as a partner it must be satisfied that he or she discharges the duties and exercises the powers of a principal in the partnership and that, unless an approved job sharer, he or she is entitled to a share of the profits based on one of the following options.

- If contracted to be available for at least 26 hours a week, a share of not less than one third of that of the partner with the greatest share.

- If contracted to be available for between 19 and 26 hours, not less than one quarter of the greatest share.
- If contracted to be available for between 13 and 19 hours, not less than one fifth of the greatest share.

If any partner's share is grossly out of line with his or her contribution to the work of the practice, a concealed sale of goodwill may be deemed to have taken place (*see* Box 2.5).

Box 2.5: A sale of goodwill is prohibited

The Medical Practices Committee (MPC) is responsible for issues concerning the sale of goodwill. Since 1948 GPs have been forbidden to sell the 'goodwill' of an NHS practice, 'goodwill' being the established custom or popularity of a practice. Examples of deemed sales of goodwill include:

- sale of premises for substantially more than might have been expected if they had not previously been used for general practice
- a significant payment other than for undertaking partnership duties
- receipt by a partner of a significantly smaller amount for his or her services than might reasonably be expected.

In particular, the MPC seeks to assure itself that the balance between profit share and workload is equitable. The MPC may consider evidence of a sale of goodwill to include:

- failure of a new partner to reach parity in the partnership profits within three years
- one or more partners being permitted to do less than a fair share of practice workload
- one or more partners getting longer or shorter holidays or, exceptionally, having an unequal entitlement to study leave
- continued restriction, after a reasonable assessment period, on a partner in taking onto his or her list any patient who chooses to register with him or her
- non-mutual terms of expulsion, retirement or dissolution.

Any GP about to join a practice, who is concerned about a possible sale of goodwill, may submit the terms of the proposed partnership to the Medical Practices Committee.

An incoming partner's share should be sufficient for it to be more than he or she might have earned as an assistant; this share should increase each year so that parity is reached within a reasonable time span (normally three years).

A written and comprehensive partnership agreement should provide equity for all partners and a reasonable level of security. Although the list sizes of individual partners should have no significance in respect of each partner's rights and obligations, it is taken as clear evidence of good faith if provision is made for a new partner to acquire a list of equal size as soon as is reasonably practicable (*see* Figure 2.5 on page 17).

Box 2.6: Discrimination is prohibited

It is unlawful for any partnership to discriminate on grounds of sex or marital status, and for a partnership of six or more to discriminate on grounds of colour, race, nationality (including citizenship), or ethnic or national origins:

- when appointing a new partner
- in the terms on which the new partner is offered a partnership
- by refusing, or deliberately neglecting, to offer a partnership;

and where someone is already a partner:

- in the way he or she is afforded access to any benefits, facilities or services
- by refusing, or deliberately neglecting, to afford access to those benefits, facilities and services
- by dismissing the partner, or treating him or her unfavourably in any other way.

Attending to the affairs of the practice

The agreement should state the time and attention which partners are expected to give to the work of the partnership, especially if one partner is allowed to give less time than others to its business. If the partners are required to devote all their time to the practice, it is useful for the agreement to stipulate that they should not engage in any other business or accept any office (eg local councillor) without the consent of the other partners.

> 'Exploitation of a junior partner'
>
> 'Dear Dr C,
> Further to your request for information on the practice's arrangements for allocating patients to each partner's list, I can confirm that patients are divided as follows:
>
> | Patients with Surname | To doctor |
> |---|---|
> | A – end of Lane | A |
> | Lapping – end of Watson | B |
> | all remaining patients | C |
>
> I hope this information is helpful.'
>
> **Figure 2.5** Extract from an FHSA General Manager's letter in the BMA files

Management of practice staff

The partnership agreement should specify who carries responsibility for staff matters. It is advisable that staff employed by the partnership should be engaged and dismissed with the consent of all partners, otherwise a dismissed employee could pursue a successful dismissal claim against the partnership as a whole. It is also essential that the agreement should prevent one partner answering or sending letters concerning employment matters without the consent of other partners. Hastily written letters often cause problems.

> 'Staff dismissal led to rift'
>
> A busy urban four-doctor partnership decided to make several significant changes in the organization of its practice staff. These included introducing a new computer system, leading to an enlarged job description for the practice manager.
> The senior receptionist was not happy about the changes and felt that the practice manager was usurping some of her work. Tension grew and came to a head when she had a blazing row with one of the partners. The latter discussed it with the other partner on duty and dismissed the

receptionist that day. When the other two partners were informed, they felt the decision had been too hasty.

The senior receptionist immediately applied to the industrial tribunal claiming unfair dismissal. Strains appeared within the partnership and it split into two before the hearing. The two partners who had not been involved in the dismissal believed they had no responsibility or financial liability with regard to the industrial tribunal case.

The tribunal found in favour of the dismissed receptionist who was awarded almost £10 000. The doctors who had not been responsible for the dismissal believed that they were not liable for the payment. However, lack of any reference in the partnership agreement to the dismissal of staff meant that all four partners were jointly responsible and liable to contribute to the damages.

Figure 2.6 A case study from the BMA files

Partnership decisions

According to the 1890 Partnership Act, differences of opinion in the partnership are settled by majority decision unless the partnership agreement specifies another arrangement. A partnership must decide whether decisions are to be taken on the basis of majority voting and, if so, what margin of majority is required to endorse a decision.

How this question is approached usually depends on partnership size. For example, in a partnership of three, the partners may opt for unanimity on all decisions. Alternatively, a partnership of six may consider that unanimity is too difficult to achieve and may consider that a majority of four to two provides a satisfactory basis for decisions. Whatever approach is adopted, this should be specified in the agreement. If there are job share partners, the agreement should specify whether they exercise a half or whole vote each.

Irrespective of how a partnership approaches routine decision making, major decisions which affect key features of the agreement should normally be taken only if there is unanimity. The nature of such decisions should be defined in the agreement.

Taxation arrangements

Each partner is jointly and severally liable for the income tax on the whole of the practice's net profits and could be sued for the whole of this amount (*see* Figure 2.7 below). In theory this is a formidable responsibility; the partnership agreement should therefore provide for enough funds to be set aside for tax liabilities, preferably in a separate bank or building society account earmarked for this purpose.

'Paying somebody else's income tax!'

Drs C, D and E were permitted to draw their full share of the profits. Each made his own arrangements to pay income tax and also indemnified the others against all such liabilities.

Dr D got into financial and marital difficulties which culminated in divorce. He is, among other things, forced to sell the matrimonial home; this enables him to meet most of his personal debts, but leaves him without further assets.

After informing his partners that he needs to get away for a while, he takes a holiday, goes abroad, and is never seen again. The Inland Revenue claim Dr D's outstanding tax from Drs C and E, who then realize that the protection they thought they had from their joint indemnities is no protection at all.

Figure 2.7 A case study from the BMA files

Under partnership law the admission or departure of a partner brings the existing partnership to an end and leads to the formation of a new partnership. However, the partners may elect to be assessed for tax on the basis that the former business has continued. This continuation election must be made within two years of the date of change and must be explicitly agreed to by all members of the 'old' and 'new' partnerships, or in the case of a deceased partner, by his or her personal representative.

It is normally advantageous to a partnership for it to elect to be taxed on a continuation basis. However, this election can increase the personal tax bills of individual partners. It is therefore preferable that the agreement requires a retiring or incoming partner to agree to a continuation election. Some partnerships indemnify a retiring or incoming partner against any additional personal tax liability resulting from it.

Holidays and study leave

Each partner should be eligible on an equitable basis for equivalent amounts of leave. If a locum is employed to cover holiday or study leave, the expenses should normally be met by the partnership as a whole. It is advisable for the agreement to restrict the number of partners who can be on leave simultaneously and the maximum length of continuous leave which can be taken.

'Surprised by holiday arrangements'

In a three partner practice, a new partner signed a partnership agreement whereby he agreed to cover holiday periods, etc. The three partners also agreed that they would cover each other's holidays to avoid the cost of hiring locums. Unfortunately for the new partner, he had neglected to take account of the fact that the other two partners were married to each other and took their holidays together. As a result, the new partner found himself providing continuous cover for the whole practice for at least six weeks each year.

Figure 2.8 A case study from the BMA files

Sickness and pregnancy

Partnerships can make various arrangements to pay for locums employed during prolonged absences. A simple method is for the absent partner to pay all the locum expenses. However, it is increasingly common for the first few weeks of locum expenses to be paid by the whole partnership.

A partnership will be infringing the 1986 Sex Discrimination Act if a pregnant partner is treated less favourably than a male partner with a male incapacity. Therefore, a partner on maternity leave should not have to meet the full cost of a locum unless this arrangement also applies to sickness leave.

Additional payments made by the FHSA or Health Board during sickness or confinement should be paid to the absent partner if he or she is responsible for locum expenses.

The question of how long the partnership or the individual partner pays locum expenses needs to be decided in relation to the arrangements for insurance cover for income protection and/or locum expenses.

Box 2.7: Recommended arrangements for maternity leave

- Fourteen weeks absence should be regarded as a minimum entitlement and the pregnant partner should have the right to determine for herself when the period of absence should start, in consultation with her own GP.

- The practice should consider the question of funding the cost of a locum to cover the actual workload of the pregnant partner, not merely her hours of availability.

- The partnership should agree on a maximum period of absence following which the partner's failure to return to work may justify compulsory expulsion from the partnership.

- The exercise of a partner's right to maternity leave should not abolish her entitlement to pro rata holiday and sickness leave.
- Where adoption is a possibility the partnership agreement should specify leave arrangements.

A partnership agreement which provides for maternity leave on terms which are less advantageous than for sick leave could be construed as evidence of indirect sex discrimination.

Leaving the partnership

The agreement should specify the conditions under which partners may leave, including the required period of notice. It is usually simpler if the period of notice expires on a quarter-day, so as to coincide with quarterly FHSA or Health Board payments. The notice itself should not be less than three months because FHSAs and Health Boards are entitled to three months' notice before removing a GP's name from the NHS medical list.

According to the 1890 Partnership Act, a partner cannot be expelled by a majority decision unless the agreement allows for this. Thus the agreement should contain a clause which makes provision for the expulsion of a partner in specific circumstances such as prolonged incapacity, mental ill-health, removal or suspension from the medical register or NHS medical list, gross breaches of the partnership agreement and bankruptcy. Although such a clause, if included, would confer a right to expel a partner in certain specific circumstances, it may, like any other clause, be waived by mutual consent.

Most partnership agreements require a partner to retire after a period of prolonged incapacity which prevents him or her from doing a fair share of the work for a period of six to 12 months. Most partnerships seek to be as generous as possible in such circumstances, but because the prolonged absence of a partner imposes a considerable burden on colleagues, it may be advisable to require an incoming partner to produce evidence of good health before the partnership agreement is signed.

Retirement

All GPs are required to retire from NHS practice by or on their 70th birthday. Thus it is sensible to include in the agreement a requirement that each partner retire from the practice by or on this compulsory retirement date. It may be advisable also to include a clause which allows a partner to continue to practise as a partner in a non-NHS capacity beyond a certain age, if the other partners agree.

However, it is normal for a partnership to agree on a retirement age below 70. A partnership should agree on a clear and fair policy on retirement before individual problems arise. Difficulties can arise if a practice only considers the issue of its retirement policy when the retirement of an individual partner is under discussion.

The issue of retirement can be particularly contentious for any partnership. Younger and older partners often express differing views on the subject, and a partner's perception of the issue may alter as he or she grows older and retirement approaches.

Restrictive covenants

NHS legislation prohibits the purchase or sale of goodwill, but not goodwill as such. Thus it is legal to protect goodwill by reasonable restrictions on the future activities of a departing partner. Such restrictions are commonplace, proper and usually enforceable, but any restraint must be entirely reasonable.

Any restrictive covenant must apply equally to all partners, relate only to work normally undertaken by a GP and should not be of excessive duration. Any restriction on working in a defined area must be reasonable; the practice should have a significant number of patients right up to the boundary and the area should not include any large concentrations of population which are of little or no significance to the practice. It may be advisable for the partnership agreement to refer to the practice area map which would normally be a reasonable area within which to restrict an outgoing partner from practising. The map itself could be included as part of the partnership agreement.

It is preferable to have a limited restraint clause which is capable of being enforced, rather than a draconian one which proves unenforceable. Moreover, it is important to note that, in recent years, courts have taken an increasingly critical view of restrictive covenants.

The Medical Practices Committee has issued important advice on restraint clauses (*see* Box 2.8), particularly in relation to the length of time and distance specified.

Defence body subscriptions

Each partner should be required to be a member of a medical defence organization or hold medical indemnity insurance whilst a member of the partnership.

> **Box 2.8: Restrictive covenants: advice from the Medical Practices Committee**
>
> - The MPC looks at restrictive covenants to see if they are reasonable and mutual in their application. If the provisions are regarded as unreasonable or too restrictive, the MPC may consider this to be evidence of a sale of goodwill.
>
> - The MPC, in forming its opinion, normally regards as an acceptable maximum a restrictive covenant which prevents a doctor engaging in NHS general practice and/or treating certain patients within a radius of two miles from the main premises for a period of two years. But variations may be justified in special circumstances.
>
> - The MPC would also consider that there might be evidence of sale of goodwill if the radius and duration were both reasonable, but the covenant included extra restrictions on a doctor acting in a capacity other than as a GP, eg if it prevented the doctor from filling a hospital appointment within the radius.

Banking arrangements

The agreement should name the partnership's bankers and should specify the arrangements for signing cheques. Normally the signatures of at least two partners should be required, either for all banking transactions or for cheques over a specific amount. (A practice manager may be one of the signatories on cheques under a specific ceiling.)

> Extract from a partnership agreement signed in 1990
>
> The partnership bank account shall be under the sole control of the principal partner and any cheque thereon shall be signed by him alone. The junior partner hereby appoints the principal partner as his attorney for all purposes in connection with the operation of the said bank account and the signing of cheques drawn thereon.
>
> Figure 2.9   An example from the BMA files

Partnership accounts

The agreement should name the partnership's accountants and the arrangements for drawing up the accounts, including the dates of the practice's financial year. It is advisable to require all partners to sign the annual accounts for them to be binding.

All partners must have free access to the partnership's accounts and records. Any denial of access to any partner is strong prima facie evidence that the doctor concerned is in fact an employee, not a partner. It may be advisable to include in the agreement a provision that all partners and their agents (eg personal accountants) should have copies of the accounts.

Arbitration

However carefully drafted, no partnership agreement can cover all contingencies; disputes and differences of opinion occur even in the most harmonious partnerships. Most of these can be resolved within the partnership, sometimes with advice or assistance from the local BMA office, or with assistance from an independent conciliator. Traditionally, the BMA has advised doctors to make provision in their partnership agreements for disputes to be referred by mutual agreement to independent arbitration. In practice, the use of arbitration should be very rare indeed. It is almost invariably an expensive process (usually far more costly than initially anticipated), more legalistic than is often assumed and, perhaps most importantly, often accompanies a final breakdown in the partnership rather than contributing to its continuation. Thus, although arbitration may be appropriate in certain specific circumstances, the extent of these is far more limited than is generally assumed.

> 'Sledgehammer to crack a nut?'
>
> In a partnership of seven, a majority of partners (6–1) decided to purchase pregnancy testing equipment to the value of £250. The one partner opposed was very unhappy with the decision. He deemed this expenditure to be unnecessary and inappropriate, believing that the provision of a pregnancy testing service would result in its use prior to abortion. He also objected to the provision of such a service free of charge. He could not prevent his partners from offering this service to their patients, but he did not see why they should be so doing at the expense of the partnership, ie partly at his own expense. The matter was referred to arbitration. The arbitration decision was lengthy and costly, and led ultimately to the dissolution of the partnership. All parties incurred several thousands of pounds of legal costs and the only outcome was a dissolution which was also costly.

Figure 2.10 A case study from the BMA files

The best advice is for all partners to consider carefully the possible consequences of any action they may be contemplating, individually or collectively, which could precipitate arbitration and lead ultimately to the dissolution of the partnership. Any type of legal action, including arbitration, is almost invariably a costly option and is, in the vast majority of cases, associated with the breakup of the partnership.

3 When Partners Fall Out: Legal Remedies

Lynne Abbess

Avoiding disputes

GOOD communication and forward planning are two key tasks which help to avoid the pitfalls of partnership life. With the pressures of practice becoming ever more paramount, it is increasingly difficult for any GP to spare the time required to 'indulge' in either of these tasks and it is tempting in the enthusiasm of the moment for a new partner to accept at face value and without question the offer of partnership, or for an existing partnership to talk itself into a new cost rent scheme. It is all too easy to enter into commitments, but 10 times more difficult, and often very costly, subsequently to extract oneself.

These days everybody's life is governed by deadlines, many of which are set for quite justifiable reasons. However, if you have endeavoured to work to a deadline which proves impossible to meet, it is usually infinitely preferable to be brave enough to admit that you are not ready to commit yourself to a particular course of action, than to allow yourself to be bounced into it only to discover later you have scored an own goal. Therefore, it is essential to seek both legal and financial advice before entering into a partnership and not simply to accept the words of reassurance from your prospective senior partner that 'everything will come out in the wash' — you do not then want to find yourself swept away on the tide!

Forward planning involves achieving as much certainty for all members of the partnership as possible. Accordingly, the more evidence of earlier agreements between the parties the better — the 'weight' of that evidence is crucial. The most obvious example of 'good evidence' is a properly drawn partnership deed. This can be supplemented by recorded minutes of partnership meetings which should be initialled by the partners in respect of those matters which might be particularly contentious within the partnership.

The weakest form of evidence is verbal evidence. GPs should never put themselves into a position where it is necessary to have to rely on verbal evidence, particularly given the complications associated with the evidential rule of 'hearsay'.

The purpose of establishing clear and solid evidence is to build a picture of the pattern of working relationships that the partners have chosen to follow. Although clear and demonstrable evidence may not prevent disputes from occurring, it can certainly help to resolve them.

Picking up the pieces

Partnership is often likened to the constitution of marriage, although it is infinitely more complex since each partner usually has more than one spouse! Inevitably, if a partnership starts to degenerate, matters can go from bad to worse very quickly and can continue on a downward spiral unless urgent steps are taken to avert disaster. Often the success of such action depends largely on the personalities of the partners. By definition, a true partnership does not lend itself to the creation of a leader, because in legal terms all partners are of equal status. Thus, no legal significance as such is attached to the term 'senior partner', and indeed it would be legally inappropriate to provide for a senior partner to have a casting vote in partnership meetings. This arrangement can be contrasted with a limited company which has a definite hierarchical structure extending downwards from the chairman and the managing director.

The first step to be taken when 'picking up the pieces' is to recognize that a real problem exists and to try to define it in clear and unambiguous terms. This is not always easily done. The next stage is to give yourselves sufficient time to discuss, and one hopes resolve, the problem in a properly constituted partnership meeting. You cannot hope to succeed in resolving the problem if you try to deal with it through hurried and ad hoc meetings amongst patients and staff during the course of the surgery routine. If necessary you should bring in a locum to cover the period of the partnership meeting to ensure that there is time for a full and frank discussion between all partners. It is usually helpful if minutes of the meeting are taken by a third party, eg your practice manager or even an independent person from outside the practice, whom you all trust. Depending upon how matters progress, further meetings may be necessary, and these in particular may be usefully chaired by an independent third party (eg a BMA industrial relations officer).

Two key principles should apply to these meetings:

- Everyone should be well prepared. If you know that certain papers need to be referred to, ensure that you have copies in advance and circulate them to the other partners; make sure they are properly indexed and you are familiar with their content. If the problem is financial, seek financial advice in advance. You may even consider it appropriate, with the consent of your partners, for the partnership accountant to be invited to attend the meeting. A similar invitation could be extended to the partnership solicitor.
- Concentrate on the future and not on the past. You are endeavouring to resolve the dispute and you must try to do so, putting the past well and truly behind you. It is rarely helpful and often highly disruptive to rehearse historical events. This tends to serve no other purpose than to put up the backs of other partners.

Above all, if the dispute is of a serious nature and it is clear that it cannot be resolved by the partnership acting on its own, do not delay in seeking independent legal advice. You may be anxious about incurring legal costs but early action can often nip a problem in the bud, thereby avoiding additional costs that might otherwise be incurred.

Partners' legal responsibilities and rights

Partners are jointly and severally liable for each other's actions. This means that one partner can bind the partnership as a whole to a course of action and a third party can pursue a claim against an individual partner, whether or not that individual was directly involved in the relationship with the third party. For example, if Drs X and Y are in partnership and Dr X orders a supply of drugs but fails to pay the invoice, the supplier can sue not only Dr X or both partners jointly, but also Dr Y as an individual. Each partner has unlimited liability (unlike the directors of a company) so that, once he or she becomes a partner of a practice, he or she exposes not only his or her share of any partnership assets but also personal assets in the event of any claim being made. This demonstrates the importance and the practical significance of the two key tasks referred to above: forward planning and good communication.

Unless a written partnership contract is entered into, the partnership will be governed by the Partnership Act 1890 which provides for the establishment of a 'partnership at will'. However, this legislation, having been enacted over a century ago, does not cater for the commercial reality of current partnerships. For example, the Partnership Act provides little comfort to a retiring partner who is trying to dispose of his or her share in the surgery premises; and if the premises have been developed under a cost rent scheme, heaven help him or her!

Although partnership legislation (such as it is) establishes the responsibilities of partners, the only satisfactory way in which partners can establish their 'rights' is to enter into a partnership contract which supplements the legislation. This contract should be completed at the earliest possible opportunity, preferably before a new partnership begins. Partners should also recognize that, even if a current contract is in existence, when a new partner is appointed to the practice, unless he or she gives express consent to be bound by the terms of the existing contract, its terms will be negated even in respect of the original partners! If this should happen, the newly formed partnership will operate as a 'partnership at will'.

Legal remedies

It could be said that the only true legal remedies are those obtained by applying to a court to enforce either 'the law' (ie Parliamentary statutes and related ensuing regulations) or a partnership agreement.

The application to a court will involve issuing a summons or writ and pursuing a quite lengthy and technical legal procedure. You may be surprised to find that it can take many months, or even years, to reach the court, and in a partnership there may be problems which simply cannot wait that long before a final decision is reached. Therefore, in certain circumstances it may be possible to apply for an interim order, eg an injunction (to prevent someone from doing something) or a mandatory injunction (to require someone to do something). These orders can give 'temporary relief' until such time as a court can consider the matter at a full hearing (often several months later).

Nobody should ever assume that court action can provide an answer to all problems. It rarely does and must be regarded as a last resort, to be undertaken only if there is no realistic alternative. Pursuing a matter through the courts is usually very costly, and even if it is successful the winning side is unlikely to recover all their costs; thus 'success' in this context can often be a pyrrhic victory. Hard as it may be to swallow, the best advice may be to agree to a compromise at a much earlier stage, long before court action is even contemplated.

Bearing this advice in mind, the court process can fulfil a useful function; the mere threat of legal proceedings can be a valuable 'negotiating tool'.

It may even be worth issuing a writ merely to show that you are serious in your intentions, whilst continuing to negotiate behind the scenes. However, you should take care to ensure that your writ does not generate an unwanted counterclaim!

In addition to strictly legal remedies, there are other methods of settling disputes, including arbitration and conciliation.

Arbitration

The term 'arbitration' is used to describe various procedures involving different levels of formality. (Technically, arbitration is defined in the Arbitration Acts of 1950 and 1979). It is usually considered to be a quick and less costly alternative to court action and arbitration clauses are often included in partnership agreements. However, experience has shown that arbitration is often neither quick nor cost effective.

Arbitration can encompass the worst of both worlds; because it does not have the formality of court proceedings it can create uncertainty in respect of both its procedure and outcome. In arbitration proceedings, it is not unusual for each party to instruct both a solicitor and barrister, and for a senior barrister to be appointed as arbitrator. The rules of evidence which govern court proceedings may not be followed strictly or even at all in arbitration proceedings, and the procedure is consequently unstructured and unsatisfactory. The cost implications can also be horrendous. In addition to the legal representatives acting for both sides, the arbitrator is also entitled to a fee; at least High Court judges are free!

Therefore, you may wish to reflect carefully before including a standard arbitration clause in your partnership agreement. Its omission does not prevent partners agreeing to proceed to arbitration if they wish to do so, but it would allow those who wanted to pursue other remedies the opportunity of doing so.

How a lawyer can assist

In most cases when partners fall out, no outside intervention or advice is required. However, if the matter is of a more serious nature, it is preferable for a lawyer to be brought in earlier rather than later.

A lawyer is often able to take the heat out of the dispute. It is usually easier for a partner to express problems freely to his or her lawyer than

Box 3.1: Case studies in partnership breakups

The following illustrates the importance of a partnership having a properly drawn contract. Drs X and Y are in partnership. Dr X discovers that Dr Y has been acting in bad faith. Contrary to the policy of the partnership, he is registering all new patients in his name and transferring some existing patients registered with Dr X to his own list without the knowledge or consent of Dr X. This, together with other factors, makes it clear that a major dispute is in the offing and Dr X therefore decides he has no alternative but to end the partnership. Dr X owns the surgery premises and Dr Y has been allowed to occupy these as a licensee free of charge (all rent reimbursement being paid to Dr X).

Scenario 1
Drs X and Y have a properly drawn partnership deed with a compulsory retirement clause which is operative if one party commits an act of bad faith. There is also a reasonable restrictive covenant which is legally enforceable.

Dr X is able to serve notice on Dr Y according to the terms of the partnership agreement, terminating the partnership forthwith. He is also able to require Dr Y to leave the surgery premises immediately and to transfer all patients on his list to that of Dr X. Should Dr Y fail to comply with this notice, Dr X could apply to the court to obtain an injunction preventing Dr Y from entering the premises and requiring him to transfer his patients to Dr X. Those patients transferred to Dr X are not obliged to remain with him, but the restrictive covenant should at least prevent them from transferring back to Dr Y within the period of restriction.

Scenario 2
Drs X and Y do not have a written agreement and are a partnership at will. Dr X serves notice on Dr Y, dissolving the partnership with immediate effect. There is no restrictive covenant and Dr Y claims that, as a licensee in the premises, he has the right to reasonable notice. Furthermore, he intends to retain his list of patients.

> **Box 3.1:** *continued*
>
> Dr X seeks to stop Dr Y from entering the premises and Dr Y applies to the court for an injunction to prevent Dr X from barring him. It is likely the court would decide that Dr Y is entitled to remain in the premises as a licensee for a minimum of three or even six months after the date of dissolution. As he is only a licensee, it would be unwise for Dr X to seek any payment from him other than his share of the running expenses (including gas, electricity, and telephone charges, but not rent). Furthermore Dr X could not seek to impose any restriction upon Dr Y to prevent him from retaining his list of patients or from acquiring an alternative list in close proximity to the surgery, and therefore he could not stop Dr Y from becoming a direct competitor.

to his or her partners directly. Moreover, the remedies available to an individual may not be immediately apparent, particularly in disputes involving premises.

A lawyer may advise that what you believe to be your moral right does not constitute a legal right. It is far better to know weaknesses in your case at the beginning, rather than to wage a battle which you have no prospect of ever winning.

If you are unfortunate enough to have to proceed to court action, you are unlikely to have either the time or the experience to handle your case properly. An experienced lawyer should know suitable 'expert witnesses' and barristers experienced in the field, if these are required.

Lawyers are also experienced in negotiations and can conduct simultaneously two 'levels' of correspondence, both 'open' and 'without prejudice', to reach a settlement. The partners themselves could not adopt this approach if conducting the case face to face.

Finally, remember that, when dealing with your lawyer, you should adopt the same principle as with your partners; the two key tasks of good communication and forward planning always achieve the best results in the end.

4 Is your Partnership Working? The Role of Mediation

Nick Gild

GPs are frequently advised to ensure that they have an up-to-date partnership agreement. Although this is obviously good advice, in fact many practices either do not have any written agreement or deed, or have one that is substantially out of date. The pace of change, even if viewed simply in terms of personnel and premises, may well have outstripped the best joint administrative efforts of the senior or managing partner and practice solicitor charged with producing or updating the partnership deed. What should you do in these circumstances? Of course, you have to make the best of a bad job. The solution does not, and should not, depend solely on interpreting and applying the legal rights and remedies of partners, but also on relationships.

Keeping the partnership healthy

Chapter 3 compared partnership to marriage; although the analogy tends to be overworked, there are genuine parallels. Marriages, like partnerships, often start to go wrong when husband and wife stop communicating effectively, not merely in major things, but also over routine and minor ones.

How can you avoid the consequences of lack of communication in partnership? Whether you have a deed or not, it is essential to construct a framework for the practice which encourages self-discipline and creates opportunities for, and the habit of, communicating with each other, both as partners in a business and as members of a clinical team.

Hold regular formal partners' meetings; keep minutes, but make sure the presence of the minute taker does not stifle free and frank discussion. If the practice manager is not the appropriate minute taker, partners should take turns to do it on the basis of a quarterly rota. The chairmanship of the meetings should also rotate amongst all the partners and the senior partner may find that his or her views, when expressed from the floor, achieve at least as much weight as when expressed from the chair. Chairing a meeting is an onerous task which often detracts from the effective exposition of one's own ideas.

Circulate draft minutes for approval within seven days after the meeting. Minor changes to the partnership deed/arrangements may be agreed at such meetings, and if duly recorded in minutes which are subsequently approved by all partners, they will be binding.

Informal contacts pay dividends too, but the right structure is needed to foster them. One option is a sandwich lunch for partners only, weekly or at least fortnightly, for which, generally, there is no agenda and partners just have the opportunity to chat. Issues directly affecting the practice or its patients may, or may not, get discussed. Such informal meetings are less about 'what?' than 'who?', and they should be aimed at cementing relations between partners which are liable to lose stability if their foundations are not maintained.

However, the practice team does not consist, by any means, of partners only. Partners and staff should meet frequently to discuss clinical and practical issues, and appearance at these meetings should be no more optional for partners than for other members of the team.

'But', I hear you cry, 'all this cementing is all very well, but what about the patients?'; and I reply that this approach to partnership practice is, at every stage, for the benefit of the patients. Some judicious timetabling in the practice now will benefit the patients far more than judicial intervention later! It will stand you in good stead financially and, if the worst should happen despite your efforts to level the playing field and give everybody some of the ball, you will find that your disciplined approach to practice has provided some prospect of ensuring that, on dissolution of your partnership, people get what they deserve.

Let us be clear, however, that a system of informal and formal meetings of partners and staff, and the keeping and agreement of minutes, whilst a foundation for a healthy practice, will do no more for an ailing practice than provide a basic framework on which to hang the ingredients of a workable dissolution. If you have reached this stage, personal relationships alone will not save the partnership. You will wish you had a modern partnership deed!

If you have no deed, and a partner is disaffected, he or she can bring disaster on your house. The next section looks at the form and extent of the disaster and some means of damage control which may be available. It also sets out a number of options, of which dissolution is only one, that are likely to be available to you if you do have a partnership deed.

What can be done if your partnership is not working?

First, let's look at the options available to a partnership with a good, modern partnership deed. Unless these can be negotiated in the heat of battle, none of them is available to the partnership which has no deed; dissolution means the immediate end of a 'partnership at will' whereas partners with a deed will at least see tomorrow dawn together.

The options include:

- voluntary retirement by a partner
- compulsory retirement (expulsion), if grounds exist
- division into two or more groups.

All the while, the partnership itself survives and is protected by its restrictive covenant. The above options exist because the fundamental tenet of a well drawn medical partnership deed is that the partnership will continue, despite the departure at various times and from various causes of some partners, for as long as at least two of the original partners remain.

This is what lawyers call a 'joint lives' partnership, which may be contrasted with a partnership for a fixed term or a partnership for the fulfilment of a single object. Neither of these latter species is likely to be appropriate to medical partnerships in the business of providing general medical services under the NHS or otherwise.

There are many admirable deeds in existence, drawn on the 'joint lives' basis, which are silent on the matter of dissolution. They contemplate only what we saw in the last paragraph, namely that while two or more are gathered together the partnership will subsist. If partners who are parties to such a deed fall out, it will preserve the assets of the practice for the benefit of those who remain, and so the patients at least will benefit.

A partnership without a deed is basically governed by the 1890 Partnership Act, which implies only the most basic of terms (*see* page 8). Such a 'partnership at will' may effectively depend for its continued existence, or not, upon the whim of one partner. It is thus highly volatile.

Volatility is the last thing partners need if they aim, as most do, to construct a solid basis for their professional lives. Partners who are opportunists or oppressors positively espouse this volatility; they either take advantage (the opportunists) by establishing themselves in a practice others have worked hard to build up and then depart the partnership with the spoils, or (if oppressors) take on partners – 'exploit' is really the word – overwork them and underpay them, and then, when they complain or show the slightest sign of character or determination, dissolve the partnership and find another innocent. Look out for these types; they are not always easy to spot until it is too late.

The fundamental volatility of the 'partnership at will' derives from those provisions of the 1890 Partnership Act which enable any one partner, at any time and without any grounds, to say to the other or others, regardless of their number, 'The partnership between us is dissolved with immediate effect'. If, instead, he were to say, 'I am leaving but you are not affected by this, as between yourselves the partnership continues', he would be wrong: one cannot retire from a 'partnership at will' and leave the partnership intact. There is no alternative to dissolution.

Volatility's partner is instability and that is what you get with the 1890 Partnership Act. Unless you agree otherwise, the Act imposes a regime of sharing profits equally; every decision falling to be made by the weight of majority (except the decision to change the nature of the business or to admit a new partner); absence of opportunity to require the resignation of a partner (even on the most compelling grounds); silence on the subject of practice premises and (as we have seen) the inevitability of dissolution, with attendant statutory taxation consequences over which you have little or no control.

So, what if you have one of these partnerships and it has had it? Is your principal aim to stay in general practice serving the patients presently on your list? What are the steps to take?

Identity your major concerns in detail and write them down. They are likely to fall under the broad headings of:

- patients on my list
- practice premises
- practice staff
- finance – capital and borrowings
- finance – income and expenditure
- finance – taxation
- partners' aims.

The last of these may not automatically occur to you, but I regard it as indispensable, so much so that it ought to head the list. Lots of people pride themselves on knowing their legal position and their so-called rights, and if they don't there are plenty of others, qualified or otherwise, who stand ready to tell them. You may have 'right of way' in particular circumstances when driving your car, but insisting on that right can kill you. So, too, can your professional career be destroyed on the dissolution of your partnership if you stand on what you regard as your 'rights'. Indeed, we have seen how few you have, and how little room there is for manoeuvre, when the relevant law is the Partnership Act 1890. This is especially so when that Act operates on dissolution in conjunction with the Income and Corporation Taxes Act 1988 and (in relation to premises) Part II of the Landlord and Tenant Act 1954 (as amended). These statutes soon become only too familiar to those embroiled in dissolution wars.

Do, therefore, try to discover what your partners want – you may be pleasantly surprised. The 56-year-old autocrat may have decided to retire at 60 and be willing to sign on the dotted line to bind himself to this; surely you can put up with him for another three or four years, particularly if he agrees that partners keep their own night visit fees and you are already doing most of those visits? The young whippersnapper is always so confrontational because he is worried about his massive borrowings, so how about parity now? Such revelations may actually save the partnership. You might have known what makes your partner tick long before things came to a head, if you had set up a system of formal and informal meetings as has been suggested in Chapter 3.

If you didn't, and dissolution has become inevitable, keep your head. Convene a formal meeting of partners and, if they insist, their legal advisers. Prepare an agenda aimed at establishing first what common ground exists and, secondly, what is not agreed but is thought fundamental by those concerned. A GP who thought he or she would have to go it alone may find that the rift is not unbridgeable with all partners; the partnership might then divide into two units. This solution provides all sorts of advantages, especially in relation to economies of scale in bearing expenses.

Whether the outcome of such a meeting is that groups form or that each partner stands alone, what will also emerge is a list of fundamental issues over which there is disagreement. Do not make the mistake of treating this as if it were an indivisible whole: aim to knock bits off it until you find out whether there is, indeed, an intractable residue. Yours may have been a partnership in which members ducked the discussion of tough subjects; break that habit now – it is not too late – and you will save yourselves grief and money.

When you are sure you have reached the intractable core of disagreement, choices present themselves; this core is, by definition, significant and has to be made to go away. Some of the means of disposing of it are potentially very expensive; namely litigation (court proceedings) and arbitration. These are particularly arid in the case of a partnership heading inevitably for dissolution, in the sense that neither the Court nor the arbitrator has any more room for manoeuvre than the parties. The Partnership Act 1890 Rules, OK? Of course not!

The need for mediation

What is needed is more, relatively informal and relatively cheap, concentration on trying to dynamite that core, yet it is plain by now that you need professional, but unbiased, help. I am sure that the answer lies in mediation and conciliation, available when the core becomes critical or much earlier. Such schemes exist in divorce and family law situations and are finding acceptance in commercial disputes. There is a place for them in partnership difficulties, and not least in the case of 'partnerships at will', where no deed exists to define issues, rights and obligations.

There is a growing recognition of the need to provide partnerships with this relatively informal assistance in resolving problems before they either become explosive or fester. I use the phrase 'relatively informal' advisedly and with two principal features in mind. The first is the importance of being able to feel that a forum exists in which one can air one's views and anxieties without destroying the partnership, and the second, not unconnected with the first, is the consequence of involving lawyers, either at all or before informal avenues for resolution have been exhausted.

It may be that medical partnerships, in contrast to those of other professionals, are particularly susceptible to breakdown or, perhaps more specifically, breakup. The provision of general medical services by principals, not assistants, is fundamental to the NHS, so doctors find themselves in partnership, and well on the way to parity of share, long before their contemporary solicitors or accountants, for example.

This means that doctors who know little about each other, either as people or practitioners, find themselves entering with breath-taking speed into the intimate relationship which partnership undoubtedly is. There may be fairly compelling grounds for saying that the interests of doctors and patients could be better served if general medical services were provided by individual GPs, each with his or her own list and allowances, joining with others only to share the expenses of practice and premises.

Whatever the preferred alternative might be, the present system is based on a type of partnership which seems to be particularly prone to serious difficulties. The comparative and frightening ease with which such a partnership blows apart may have a lot to do with the reasonable certainty felt by an established doctor that he or she will still have patients after a breakup. This may be contrasted with the dissolution of a partnership of solicitors, in the event of which no individual former partner can feel sure of any particular section of the goodwill of the former firm, ie of clients sticking with him or her.

GPs, it seems, have particular need of early help, in the form of conciliation or mediation, quite distinct in its aims from arbitration or court proceedings. Such help should, although needing a framework to incorporate the mediator's role, be essentially informal, inexpensive (compared to arbitration or court proceedings), exploratory and advisory rather than legally binding. There are several forms that this informal intervention might take and what follows is a description of one of them.

The parties choose the questions for consideration by the mediator; he or she cannot give a judgement or make a final order binding on the parties by law. The mediator would decide how to deal with the issues; he or she would be likely to hear the parties together and then talk to them privately in separate rooms. He or she would pass between them, indicating how near a settlement might be on a particular issue and stating his or her own objective view. The mediator would be experienced in the particular issues facing the partnership. At the end of the process, the parties would decide if they wanted to adopt the solution the mediator proposed, or any part of it, but they would not be obliged to do so. The cost, which would be a fraction of the cost of litigation or arbitration, would be borne in partnership shares – no question of all of it falling on the 'loser' as there would be none. Even if the mediator's proposed solution were not adopted, the process would at least have given food for thought.

5 Partnership Accounts

Valerie Martin

Introduction

Partnership accounts provide a crucial record of a practice's profit for the accounting year and show its financial worth on the balance sheet date. They also provide the Inland Revenue with information on which it assesses the tax due from the partnership. Most importantly, the accounts should enable the partners to review the practice's performance and to plan its future development. They must therefore summarize clearly and concisely the practice's income and expenses and its net worth, and provide enough information to enable partners to analyse its performance, including making comparisons with GPs' intended average gross and average net remuneration.

The income and expenditure account

This summarizes income — including investment income — and expenditure for the year. It is helpful to include the previous year's figures as comparatives so that partners can readily compare these with this year's performance.

The following principles should be followed when preparing partnership accounts.

The grossing-up principle

As the Review Body pay award takes account of the level of expenses shown in GPs' accounts, together with personal claims for expenses and business interest relief included in their tax returns, it is important that expenses are shown gross in the accounts. The NHS General Medical Services Statement of Fees and Allowances (the Red Book) advises that all income and expenses should be shown gross in the accounts, and that, for example, staff costs should not be netted off against staff reimbursements, or premises costs against rent and rates reimbursements.

The accruals basis

The income and expenditure account should be prepared on an accruals basis, ie in a way which reflects actual income earned and expenditure incurred during the accounting period, rather than simply cash paid out and received. This is particularly relevant to any partnership where there has been a change of partners or profit shares; in these circumstances it is essential that all income earned and expenditure incurred by the partners in the year is allocated between them in that year's accounts. The term 'debtors' refers to the amount of money due to the practice at the balance sheet date; this mainly consists of FHSA payments due to the practice at the end of the accounting year. For example, if the accounting year ends on 30 June, the June quarter payment should be included under the heading 'debtors' and also any fees and allowances received in the September quarter payment, which nevertheless relate to money earned during the June quarter.

Valuing drugs

A stocktake needs to be made at the end of the accounting year of all drugs held by the practice. These should be valued at either their cost or net realizable value, whichever is lower. Their value should be included in the balance sheet as an asset, being a part of the practice's net worth. Thus, if a partner retires from the practice, he or she has a share in the practice's stock of drugs as valued at the end of the accounting year.

Depreciation

This charge is included in the income and expenditure account to enable the original cost of an asset to be spread over its useful life. The appropriate proportion of the original cost of an asset should be included in the expenses for each year, rather than reducing the profit of the year of actual purchase by the whole amount of its original cost. The partners (on the advice of their accountants) should decide which depreciation rates to apply to their assets. Once these have been decided, they should be applied consistently. The following depreciation rates are commonly used:

- computer equipment $33\frac{1}{3}$% per annum
- medical equipment   20% per annum
- furniture and fittings   10% per annum
- office equipment   20% per annum
- surgery premises   not normally depreciated.

Since practices can choose their own depreciation rates, the Inland Revenue does not give tax relief on the amount of depreciation included in the accounts. Instead, it allows tax relief on the purchase of fixed assets by means of standardized capital allowances.

Allocating profits to partners

When the profit for the accounting period has been calculated, it is then distributed among the partners according to the practice's profit sharing arrangements. If there are no changes in either the partnership or its profit sharing ratios during the year, this should be a comparatively straightforward exercise. However, if such changes have occurred, it is necessary to allocate the profit by reference to the various profit sharing periods. This may be done by attempting to allocate it accurately between the different profit sharing periods, such that income earned and expenditure incurred in these periods is identified and attributed to the relevant periods. Alternatively these may be apportioned on a time basis which means that, if a new partner is admitted half-way through a year, half of the profits would be allocated to the first period and half to the second.

Obviously if the appointment or retirement of a partner is likely to affect significantly the practice's profitability, it may be advisable to apportion the income on a best estimate of the actual basis. However, it is often extremely difficult to allocate expenses on a strictly actual basis, and it may be fairer (and certainly much simpler) to apportion expenses on a time basis.

In principle, all items of practice income and expenditure must be included in the accounts so that the profit accurately reflects what is actually being generated by the practice. However, some practices have agreed that not all income should be shared among the partners according to their profit sharing ratios. Instead, income from sources such as the seniority allowance, night visit fees and the postgraduate education allowance may be retained on a personal basis by individual partners. According to this arrangement, such income should be regarded as prior shares of income and therefore allocated to partners before the resulting balance is divided between them according to the agreed profit sharing ratios. Similarly, if not all partners own the premises, or partners own the premises in different ratios to those applying to profit shares, income and expenditure relating to ownership of the surgery should be allocated as a prior charge among the property owning partners according to the ratios in which they own the premises. The net surgery income comprises FHSA rent reimbursements less interest on partnership loans relating to the premises, and any other expenditure which it is agreed should be borne by the property owning partners.

Capital grants

If FHSA improvement grants and fundholding management allowances are paid to a practice as a contribution towards its capital expenditure, these should be offset in the accounts against the cost of the relevant assets, so that only the net cost is depreciated and included in the balance sheet.

FHSA improvement grant payments and fundholding management allowances need to be shown separately as, although capital allowances may be claimed if a management allowance is paid, these cannot be claimed if an improvement grant is paid towards the cost of an asset.

Presenting the accounts

Figure 5.1 shows an example of how to lay out income and expenditure accounts for a GP practice and how to allocate profits among partners. The notes to the accounts refer partners to more detailed information so that they can analyse the practice's performance. The various NHS fees and allowances received by the practice are shown in Figure 5.2.

The practice's NHS income consists of four main elements: practice allowances, capitation payments, sessional payments and item of service fees. On average, a GP's income is distributed among these as follows:

practice allowances	20%
capitation payments	61%
sessional payments	5%
item of service fees	14%
Total	100%

DR CROSBY & PARTNERS
INCOME AND EXPENDITURE ACCOUNT
YEAR ENDED 30 JUNE 1993

	Notes	1993 £	1993 £	1992 £	1992 £
Income					
National Health Service fees	2	211 961		176 925	
Reimbursements	3	148 511		108 985	
Appointments	4	10 151		12 866	
Other income	5	10 113		7471	
Fundholding management allowance	6	24 916		12 646	
Total income			405 652		318 893
Expenditure					
Practice expenses	7		21 269		17 760
Premises expenses	7		8359		6857
Staff expenses	7		132 956		102 977
Administration expenses	7		14 622		11 206
Finance expenses	7		17 519		20 355
Depreciation			2311		1178
Fundholding expenses	6		24 916		11 168
Total expenditure			221 952		171 501
			183 700		147 392
Investment income					
Bank interest receivable			766		211
Building society interest receivable			1722		2101
			2488		2312
Net profit for the year			186 188		149 704

Allocation of profits

	Prior shares £	Share of balance £	1993 Total £	1992 Total £
Dr Crosby	11 063	38 241	49 304	41 603
Dr Stills	10 814	38 240	49 054	41 056
Dr Nash	6523	38 240	44 763	35 428
Dr Young	6791	36 726	43 067	31 617
	35 191	151 447	186 188	149 704

Figure 5.1 A sample income and expenditure account, showing allocation of profits

DR CROSBY & PARTNERS
NOTES TO THE ACCOUNTS
YEAR ENDED 30 JUNE 1993

2. National health service fees

	1993 £	1992 £
Allowances		
Practice allowances	22 835	21 732
Seniority	4900	3523
Postgraduate education allowance	8100	7727
Rural practice payments	428	308
Trainee supervision grant	4237	4021
	40 500	37 311
Capitation payments		
Capitation fees	94 237	83 673
Deprivation payments	5421	3987
Registration fees	3974	1864
Child health surveillance	5394	1142
Homeless and rootless payments	1200	924
Target payments:		
Cervical cytology	7789	6242
Childhood immunizations	6279	6566
Pre-school boosters	2330	1643
	126 624	106 041
Sessional payments		
Health promotion clinics	16 560	10 928
Minor surgery	1000	–
Teaching medical students	854	265
	18 414	11 193
Item of service fees		
Night visits	6531	5468
Temporary residents	1453	1215
Contraceptive services	5197	4217
Emergency treatment and INT	155	22
Maternity	8926	7092
Vaccinations and immunizations	4201	4366
	26 423	22 380
Total	211 961	176 925

Figure 5.2 Fees and allowances received by a practice

Partnerships should review how their income is distributed. A significant variation from the pattern shown on page 46 may point to areas where a practice can increase activity and income.

GPs are self-employed individuals for tax purposes and enter into a contract for services with their FHSAs. The Review Body's pay award sets the levels of various NHS fees and allowances for the year. It also determines the intended average gross remuneration and the element of that gross income which is deemed to cover indirect expenses, thereby arriving at a figure for intended average net remuneration. The intended gross and net income per principal as set by the Review Body are published in the medical press, and practices should compare their accounts with these intended average levels.

Direct reimbursement

In addition to receiving indirect reimbursements for general expenses through the generality of fees and allowances, GPs are also directly reimbursed for practice staff, surgery premises, computers, drugs, trainee salaries, staff training and certain locum fees. It is important that these direct reimbursements are shown clearly in the accounts so that a practice can identify easily the real cost of various activities; eg the real cost of taking on an additional member of staff is total cost less any direct reimbursement. It is essential that direct reimbursements are not netted out against expenditure, because this reduces the total amount of expenses reported to the Review Body to enable it to determine GPs' pay.

Accounting records

The information in the income and expenditure account is obtained by the practice's accountants from the practice's own accounting records. These should comprise both a cash book and a book which includes an analysis of FHSA income. The latter should summarize all fees and allowances received from the FHSA during the year, dividing them into the elements shown in Figure 5.2. This provides a vital record for the practice to monitor NHS income and quickly identify any fall below the expected level.

The balance sheet

This is a statement of the practice's financial position at the end of the accounting year. It is important to note that it is merely a snap-shot of the amounts owed to and by the practice at a particular point in time. On the very next day, cash may be received from a debtor, thereby increasing the amount shown as cash and reducing that shown as debtors, and in turn this cash may be used to pay a creditor. Such cash movements would not affect the practice's overall total net assets, although these will change during the following year as profit is earned and drawn by partners.

The balance sheet has two distinct purposes: firstly, to ascertain whether the assets of the practice are sufficient to cover its liabilities, and secondly to calculate the value of the partners' investment in the practice.

It is important to recognize that the accounts being prepared are those of the business in its own right and not those of its owners who are the partners. This is an important distinction; these have to be seen as separate entities if their relationship (which is clearly shown in the balance sheet) is to be properly understood. Partners invest their funds in the practice as a business and therefore the balance sheet shows in the capital and current accounts the amount of the funds due to the partners.

Thus the balance sheet contains:

- assets
- liabilities
- partners' funds.

Accordingly, the net assets of the partnership, which comprise its assets less its liabilities, always equal the partners' funds; thus the two halves of the balance sheet literally balance. Figure 5.3 shows how the balance sheet distinguishes between partners' funds and the use of these for different purposes. The various subheadings within 'employment of funds' are described below.

The difference between fixed and current assets

An asset may be defined as something owned by the business and available for its future use.

Fixed assets are those used by the business over a period of several years to earn profits, but which are not actually available for resale. These are depreciated to spread their cost over their working life and to apportion the cost (as far as possible) appropriately among the relevant partners.

Conversely, current assets are acquired for sale and conversion into cash during the normal course of the practice's business; eg dispensing drugs are acquired for resale to generate profit.

DR CROSBY & PARTNERS
BALANCE SHEET
YEAR ENDED 30 JUNE 1993

	Notes	1993 £	1993 £	1992 £	1992 £
Partners' funds and tax provision					
Property capital accounts	8		106 550		100 813
Capital accounts	9		20 000		20 000
Current accounts	10		4090		6211
Taxation provisions	11		15 819		14 608
			146 459		141 632
Employment of funds					
Fixed assets	13		359 363		325 260
Current assets					
Stock of drugs		621		712	
Debtors		32 180		26 956	
Balance at building society		12 271		3479	
Cash at bank and in hand		511		8769	
		45 583		39 916	
Current liabilities					
Bank overdraft		1211		–	
Creditors		13 210		9972	
Due to former partners		597		2638	
GPFC loan		6000		–	
		21 018		12 610	
Net current assets			24 565		27 306
			383 928		352 566
Long-term liabilities					
Mortgage loans			237 469		210 934
Net assets			146 459		141 632

Figure 5.3 Division of partners' funds

The term 'debtors' is used to describe monies owed to the practice for goods or services already provided which are convertible into cash, which is itself a current asset.

The difference between current and long-term liabilities

Current liabilities are amounts owed by the practice and payable within 12 months of the end of the accounting year. These include trade creditors, amounts due to former partners, capital repayments of a long-term loan due within the next 12 months, and bank overdrafts, which are always repayable on demand!

Long-term liabilities are capital amounts outstanding on loans which are repayable over a period longer than 12 months.

The total obtained by subtracting liabilities from assets is the partnership's net assets; this figure represents the net worth of the business and is equal to the partners' funds, being their investment in the practice.

Partners' funds

It assists understanding the extent of their investment in the practice if the partners' funds are divided between long-term investments (which can only be withdrawn when they retire from the practice) and those amounts which reflect the difference between partners' profit shares for the year and their drawings from the practice. The latter represents the money which may be withdrawn from the practice when the accounts are finally agreed.

Thus the partners' funds should be divided into four categories:

- property capital accounts
- capital accounts
- current accounts
- taxation provisions.

The property capital account

This is the partners' equity in the premises and is the difference between the premises cost or valuation and any outstanding partnership loans.

If the premises are funded by individual partners' personal loans rather than by a partnership loan, the property capital accounts should show the value of the premises and the partners' borrowing will be shown 'off' the balance sheet. Personal loans may be preferred to a partnership loan because tax relief on the interest is claimed on an actual year basis through partners' individual tax returns, rather than on a preceding year basis as it would be if included in the practice accounts (*see* Chapter 6).

Capital accounts

The partners' capital accounts refer to the funds provided for working capital to enable the practice to run smoothly. The amount of this working capital varies between practices, reflecting the net book value of fixed assets (excluding premises) funded by the partners rather than by partnership loans, and also the value of debtors and creditors to the practice. The capital accounts therefore fund the purchase of fixed assets and the practice's day to day expenditure, so that it can run without the risk of incurring an overdraft at times when income may be lower than expenditure.

The capital accounts should be established in the partners' profit sharing ratios to ensure that capital funding is on an equitable basis. A partner's share of this capital will remain in the practice until he or she leaves the partnership.

Current accounts

These reflect the difference between partners' share of the profits for the year less the amount they have drawn, superannuation payments and any sum earmarked for tax. Figure 5.4 shows the information which should be included to allow each partner to analyse movements in the current account during the year.

Leave advances are included in the current accounts if these are withdrawn by the partners. They are effectively interest free loans repayable by deduction from the FHSA's quarterly payments, and they therefore do not affect a practice's profit. However, if leave advances are retained by the partnership as working capital, they should not be shown in the partners' current accounts. Any amount retained at the end of the year should then be included in creditors in the balance sheet.

DR CROSBY & PARTNERS
NOTES TO THE ACCOUNTS
YEAR ENDED 30 JUNE 1993

10. Partners' current accounts

	Dr Crosby £	Dr Stills £	Dr Nash £	Dr Young £	Total £
Balance at 1 July 1992	1011	2196	1976	1028	6211
Profit for the year	49 304	49 054	44 736	43 067	186 188
Leave advances	1277	1277	1277	1277	5108
Cash introduced	210	–	–	–	210
Income tax repaid	971	1134	56	–	2161
	52 773	53 661	48 072	45 372	199 878
Monthly drawings	29 914	26 699	27 886	28 719	113 218
Fees retained privately	681	315	100	750	1846
Payment of personal expenses	210	–	–	195	405
Wives' salaries	2521	2422	2456	–	7399
Leave payments withdrawn	1277	1277	1277	1277	5108
Prior shares withdrawn	6525	6662	2025	2025	17 237
Transfers to property capital accounts (note 8)	1434	1435	1434	1434	5737
Transfers to tax provisions (note 11)	5829	6639	7121	5111	24 700
PAYE on appointments	–	1211	519	519	2249
Class 1 NIC	–	283	127	127	537
Class 2 NIC	252	252	252	252	1008
Superannuation:					
Standard	2569	2411	2201	2032	9213
Added years – variable	–	1211	576	–	1787
Appointments	–	572	–	572	1144
Leave advances repaid	1050	1050	1050	1505	4200
	52 262	52 439	47 024	44 063	195 788
Balance at 30 June 1993	511	1222	1048	1309	4090

Figure 5.4 Partners' current accounts

Providing for tax liabilities

The concept of sharing in joint and several liabilities can cause problems. At least with the partnership tax liability, the risk of having to pay a fellow partner's share of tax can be avoided by retaining within the practice the partnership tax which is due to be paid.

Making provision for tax payments is essentially a book-keeping exercise; within the practice's accounts certain amounts are charged to each partner's current account and credited to a tax provision account in the same partner's name. Payments to the Inland Revenue are drawn from these tax provision accounts. This does not necessarily require the tax to be deposited in a separate bank or building society account; it simply retains the cash in the partnership by preventing partners from withdrawing it from their current accounts. This retained money can be used by the practice as working capital, particularly since it is comparatively easy to plan in advance for its payment to the Inland Revenue.

This arrangement has the advantage of ensuring that, when a partner leaves the practice, there is no need to ask him or her to contribute to the partnership's tax liability. It is advisable to ensure that the amount set aside is sufficient to meet the preceding year tax liability up to the date of the balance sheet; thus a retiring partner should leave sufficient funds in the partnership to cover his or her share of the tax liability. So long as partners' drawings are calculated on a 'net of tax' basis, there should always be enough funds in the tax provision account to meet a partner's share of the tax liability, regardless of when a partner retires or indeed dies in service.

To illustrate this, the amount of tax provision in the accounts for the year ended 30 June 1993 should be sufficient to cover the whole of the 1992/93 liability and any earlier years not yet finally settled, and also one quarter of the 1993/94 tax liability for the period from 6 April to 30 June 1993.

Since the tax liability for the whole of the current year and the next fiscal year (being based on the current year's accounts) is known, it is helpful for partners to be given information concerning it so that they can plan their personal cash flow.

Figure 5.5 illustrates a partnership taxation provision and movements within the individual partners' tax provision accounts are shown in Figure 5.6.

Fundholding and partnership accounts

Fundholders have to produce a separate account for their fundholding activities and these must be drawn up to 31 March each year, regardless

DR CROSBY & PARTNERS
NOTES TO THE ACCOUNTS
YEAR ENDED 30 JUNE 1993

11. Partnership taxation provision

Assuming the practice continues to pay income tax on a preceding year basis and at current rates of tax, provision has been made in the accounts for the year for income tax and Class 4 NIC liabilities up to 30 June 1993.

	£
1991/92 estimated repayment due	(1393)
1992/93 balance of liability	14 854
1993/94 on preceding year basis for the period 6 April 1993–30 June 1993	2358
	15 819

The 1993/94 income tax and Class 4 NIC liabilities (against which £2358 has been provided) are estimated to be:

	£
1993/94 due 1 January 1994	4750
due 1 July 1994	4750
	9500

No provision has been made in these accounts for 1994/95 income tax and Class 4 NIC liabilities (which are based on results to 30 June 1993) which are estimated to be:

	£
1994/95 due 1 January 1995	7500
due 1 July 1995	7500
	15 000

Figure 5.5 A partnership tax provision

DR CROSBY & PARTNERS
NOTES TO THE ACCOUNTS
YEAR ENDED 30 JUNE 1993

12. Movements on taxation provision

	Dr Crosby £	Dr Stills £	Dr Nash £	Dr Young £	Subtotal £	Payments on account £	Total £
Provision brought forward at 1 July 1992	12 124	10 457	13 194	11 122	46 897	(32 289)	14 608
Charge/(release) for:							
1991/92	(1173)	40	(1020)	(5)	(2158)		(2158)
1992/93	6381	6088	7832	4199	24 500		24 500
1993/94	621	511	309	917	2358		2358
Total charge for year	5829	6639	7121	5111	24 700		24 700
(Paid)/repaid during year for:							
1991/92						(11 449)	(11 449)
1992/93						(12 040)	(12 040)
Total payment						(23 489)	(23 489)
Allocation of payment for:							
1990/91	(5013)	(6616)	(6884)	(4738)	(23 251)	23 251	–
Provision carried forward	12 940	10 480	13 431	11 495	48 346	(32 527)	15 819
Representing:							
1991/92	5598	4047	6055	3394	19 094	(20 487)	(1393)
1992/93	6721	5922	7067	7184	26 894	(12 040)	14 854
1993/94	621	511	309	917	2358	–	2358
	12 940	10 480	13 431	11 495	48 346	(32 527)	15 819

Figure 5.6 Movements on partners' tax provision accounts

of the accounting year of the main practice account. However, there is some interaction between the fundholding and main practice accounts.

The management allowance

This is paid to a practice to cover fundholding management expenses. Thus, in both the preparatory year and the fundholding years, the allowance and its related expenditure must be shown as separate items in the income and expenditure account if it is used to pay for revenue expense items. This ensures that the expenditure is grossed up for Review Body purposes.

Reimbursement of capital expenditure, both out of the management allowance and from the savings account, should be shown in the same way as grants in the fixed asset note to the accounts, thus reducing the cost of the assets to the amount contributed by the practice. In most cases this will be nil. However, capital allowances may be claimed on any net amount contributed to the cost of the assets by the practice.

The fundholding bank account

Funds held in this account are not owned by a practice's partners and therefore the account should be clearly annotated by the bank as a fundholding account. This bank account should not be referred to in the practice balance sheet. Any interest charged on it should be paid from the management allowance. The partners are not entitled to any interest on the fundholding account; it must be paid to the FHSA. Therefore, it should not be shown as income in the partnership accounts or in partners' personal tax returns.

Practice staff reimbursement

Reimbursement out of the fundholding staff fund to the partnership must be included in the practice accounts as practice staff refunds, and care should be taken to ensure that all monies due at the year end are included. If too much or too little cash has been transferred from the fundholding bank account, a balance will appear on the fundholding balance sheet as either a debtor or creditor under the heading of general practice account, and an equal and opposite entry should appear in the partnership balance sheet.

Figure 5.7 shows the note which should appear in the partnership accounts summarizing the expenditure from the fundholding management

DR CROSBY & PARTNERS
NOTES TO THE ACCOUNTS
YEAR ENDED 30 JUNE 1993

6. Fundholding management allowance

	1993 £	1992 £
Allowance received for capital assets	8084	2350
Allowance received for revenue expenditure	24 916	12 646
	33 000	14 996
Capital expenditure		
Computer equipment	6619	–
Medical equipment	1215	1454
Furniture and fittings	250	896
	8084	2350
Revenue expenditure		
Staff	17 456	5432
Locum payments	2200	2000
Training	2468	1851
Computer costs and maintenance	1246	563
Accountancy	1546	1176
Other	–	146
	24 916	11 168
Net income	–	1487

Figure 5.7 Summary of expenditure from the fundholding management allowance

allowance and the allowance received. It will be seen that the allowance received in respect of revenue items totals £24 916, and the relevant expenditure is shown in the income and expenditure account in Figure 5.1. The allowance received to reimburse capital acquisitions totals £8084, and will be set off against the cost of those items in the fixed assets note, thereby reducing the value of those fixed assets in the balance sheet.

Partners' personal expenses

Partners' personal expenses, such as the cost of running cars, can be shown in either the partnership accounts or claimed against tax on a personal expenses claim form.

The Inland Revenue treats the assessable profits for GPs as being the profit as shown in the accounts less the total of the partners' personal expense claims for the same period. Therefore the way in which these expenses are treated does not affect either the timing or the level of tax relief allowed.

Similarly, the Review Body includes partners' personal expense claims in their calculation of total expenses, and again there is no difference between claiming the expenses through the practice accounts or as personal expenses. It is important to note that under the new tax system, expenses and capital allowances will only be able to be claimed on the partnership return. It will therefore be necessary for partners to disclose their personal expenses and capital allowances to their partners so that they can be incorporated in the partnership return.

The treatment chosen should be that which is most equitable between the partners. If expenses are incurred by all partners at a similar level, they may be included in the partnership accounts without the risk of one partner bearing another's expenses.

However, if there is any element of personal choice which could affect expense levels, it is much fairer to regard personal expenditure as being paid out of that partner's profit share and tax relief should be claimed as a personal expense. Cars are probably the best example of this kind of expenditure; partners usually prefer to buy cars costing significantly different amounts and have widely differing levels of private usage.

The proportion of allowable motoring costs is based on the business usage proportion; so if a partner is able to claim 80% of usage as business usage, this proportion of motoring costs will be eligible for tax relief. Capital allowances are available on the car irrespective of whether it is owned by the partnership or the partner, and the same rules apply.

Examples of business expenses frequently claimed as personal expenses include:

- surgery facilities in private homes
- home study facilities
- medical books and journals
- courses and conferences
- home telephone bills
- laundry and cleaning
- spouse's salary for telephone answering, secretarial and counselling services.

6 Partnership Taxation

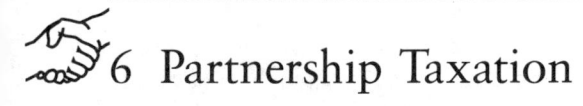

Valerie Martin

Introduction

GPs have a contract for services with the National Health Service rather than a contract of service. They are therefore self-employed individuals for tax purposes and taxed according to the rules of Schedule D.

Calculating taxable profits

The annual accounts of a practice show the net profits earned during the year and these are calculated by deducting total expenditure from total income. However, an adjustment usually has to be made to the net profits to obtain the practice's taxable profits. This is because the accounts may include expenditure which the Inland Revenue does not regard as an allowable business expense; for example, the cost of entertainment, capital expense such as legal fees relating to a new surgery, the element of personal use of any type of expenditure, interest charged by the Inland Revenue on late payment of tax, and depreciation. Depreciation is disallowed because a practice may choose to depreciate its fixed assets at any rate ranging from, say, 100% in the first year to 10% per annum.

Capital allowances

Although the Inland Revenue disallows any depreciation charged in the accounts, it does allow tax relief through a system of capital allowances which provides for a standardized rate of depreciation of 25% per annum on a reducing balance basis. If the expenditure includes an element of private use, the capital allowance is limited to that proportion which can be attributed to strictly business use. In the case of cars, the cost on which the capital allowance is calculated is restricted to £12 000 for cars purchased after 10 March 1992 and £8000 for those purchased prior to that date. When a car is sold, a balancing allowance is allowed if the tax relief so far allowed does not cover the net cost of the car (the difference between original purchase price and second hand sale price). A balancing charge may be made if too much tax relief has already been allowed (*see* Figure 6.1).

A GP purchases a car for £13 000 on 1 April 1992 and claims 80% business usage.

		£		Writing down allowance £
Year 1	Cost	13 000		
	WDA – restricted 25% × 12 000	(3000)	× 80%	2400
		10 000		
Year 2	WDA at 25%	(2500)	× 80%	2000
		7500		
Year 3	WDA at 25%	(1875)	× 80%	1500
		5625		
Year 4	Sale proceeds	(5000)		
		625		
	Balancing allowance	625	× 80%	500
		Nil		

Figure 6.1 Capital allowances on cars

It should be noted that there was a special 40% first year allowance on new assets (excluding cars) bought between 1 November 1992 and 31 October 1993. This replaced the 25% writing down allowance normally claimed in the year of purchase.

The final adjustment that needs to be made to the profits shown in the accounts, to calculate the profit assessable for tax, is to deduct any income which is either non-taxable (eg a repayment of overpaid tax) or assessed on the individual partners' tax returns under a separate assessment (eg bank or building society interest, or rental income). However, the rent reimbursement, or cost/notional rent received from the FHSA should not be deducted as rental income because this is part of the practice profits taxable under Schedule D. Further adjustment should be made to allow for any income received from other appointments, which has been already taxed at source under PAYE.

Personal expense claims

The Inland Revenue considers the taxable profit of a practice to be the tax adjusted profit as shown in its accounts, less the partnership capital allowances, partners' personal tax claims, and any other personal capital allowances applying to that period.

Therefore, it does not affect either the amount or the timing of the tax relief, whether expenses are included in the practice accounts or claimed individually through partners' personal expense claims. It is preferable to claim any expense which varies between partners through their personal expense claims rather than through the practice accounts. This ensures that partners are not subsidizing each others' expenses, particularly those relating to cars where the purchase price and running costs may vary greatly between partners. It applies also to those expenses which are not necessarily incurred by all partners, eg spouses' salaries for secretarial and telephone answering services.

Allocating the assessable profit

Having calculated the assessable profit, the next step is to allocate it between the partners according to the profit sharing ratios prevailing during the tax year in which the profit is assessed, and not according to the ratios applicable to the period when the profits were actually earned. This crucial distinction between earning profits and paying tax on them can be particularly confusing. To ensure that partners obtain tax relief on their own personal expenses and personal capital allowances, it is preferable to treat these as a prior expense of the individuals, in the same way that any income (such as seniority allowances) which is retained by individual partners is treated as a prior share of the profits.

These amounts can then be allocated to the individual partners before the balance of the assessable profit is allocated between them according to the profit sharing ratios appertaining to the tax year.

Calculating the tax liability

When the assessment has been allocated between partners it is necessary to look at each partner's individual tax position to calculate the tax payable. The following should be deducted from each individual partner's share in respect of the actual tax year:

- any personal allowances and reliefs
- personal pension premiums and superannuation
- interest on loans qualifying for tax relief.

The income tax rates for each partner are then applied to his or her share of the net taxable profit to calculate income tax and Class 4 NIC liabilities.

Joint and several liability

Having calculated each individual's income tax and Class 4 NIC liabilities, these are then added together to obtain the partnership tax liability. The Inland Revenue then issues a single assessment on the whole partnership for the total tax and Class 4 NIC due. This is because the partners have joint and several liability for the partnership tax.

The Inland Revenue requires the partnership to pay the tax, not the individual partners. This is why it is advisable for every partnership to plan for the amount of tax due to be retained by the partnership so that there is no risk of a partner being unable to meet his or her share of the joint liability.

This concept of joint and several liability for tax will cease on the introduction of the new current year basis of tax.

Preceding year basis of assessment

Under the present tax system profits of partnerships and sole practitioners are taxed on what is known as a preceding year basis; ie the assessment for a tax year is based on the profits of the accounting period ending in the previous tax year. For example, if the annual accounts are for a period ending on 31 March 1993, which is in the tax year 1992/93, the profits will be assessed in the 1993/94 tax year (*see* Figure 6.2). However, if accounts are for the year ending 30 April 1993, because this ends in the tax year 1993/94 the profits will be assessed in 1994/95 (*see* Figure 6.3).

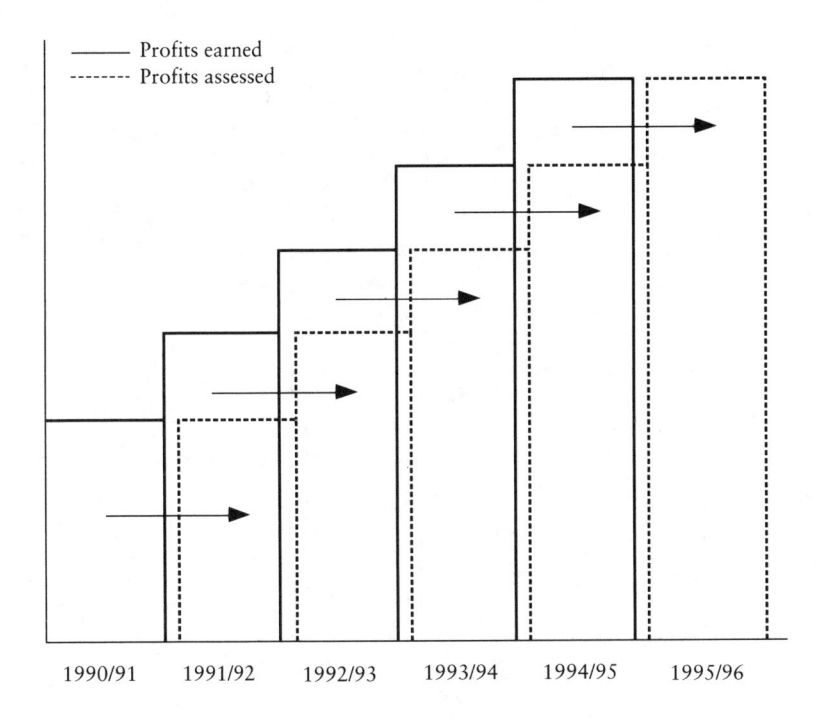

Figure 6.2 Profits assessable under the preceding year basis of assessment, accounting year end 31 March

If profits are continuing to rise, it is preferable to choose an accounting year ending early in the tax year in order to extend the period between earning profits and paying tax on them. This is why 30 April is the ideal year end date for most self-employed people. However, for GPs it is convenient to have a date coterminous with an FHSA quarter day; 30 June is therefore the optimum date, being the first quarter day after 6 April, when the tax year begins.

A case has been made for GPs to use 31 March as the end date of their accounting year because the Doctors' and Dentists' Review Body bases its expenses evidence on anonymized samples of GPs' tax returns drawn from practices whose accounting years end on 31 March. However, the BMA's General Medical Services Committee recognizes that many GPs are now using the most tax advantageous year end date and it is therefore

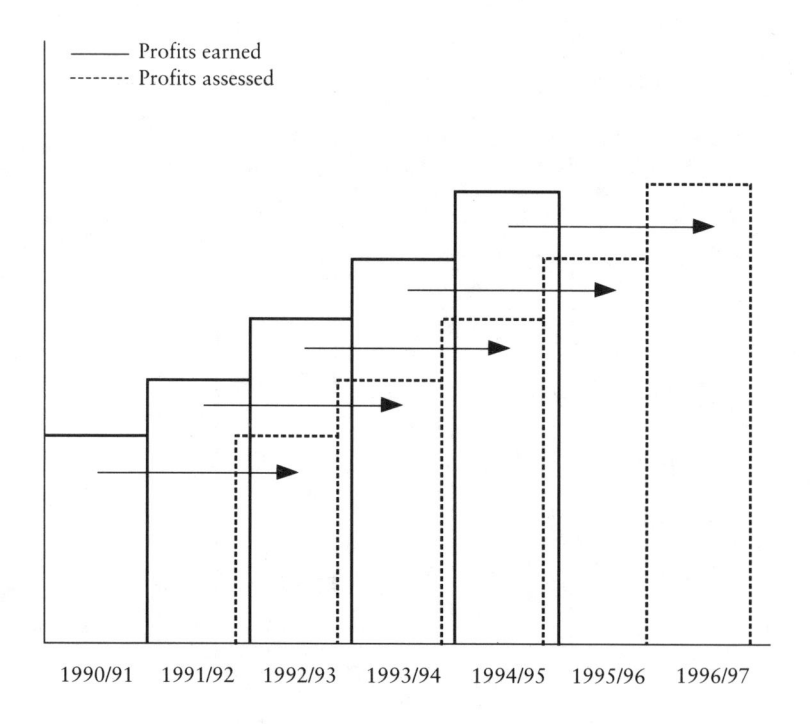

Figure 6.3 Profits assessable under the preceding year basis of assessment, accounting year end 30 April

considering how the sample survey might be changed to include practices with other accounting year end dates.

The cash flow advantage of the optimum choice of accounting year end can be seen in Figures 6.2 and 6.3. Furthermore, a retiring partner can benefit from receiving an additional slice of tax-free income: the difference between actual profits earned and profits assessed in the last two years of partnership, if a continuation election has been made.

Taxing a new partnership

Tax assessment on a normal preceding year basis lags between one and two years behind the period when profits are earned. This arrangement cannot apply at the start of a new practice, so special 'opening' year rules then apply.

- The first year is assessed on actual profits earned from the start of the partnership to the following 5 April.
- The second year is assessed on profits earned in the first 12 months.
- The third year is assessed on profits earned in the accounting year ending in the immediately preceding tax year (ie the normal preceding year basis begins to apply).

For example, if a practice commences on 1 July 1993, the opening year assessments will be:

1993/94 actual profits earned from 1 July 1993 to 5 April 1994

1994/95 profits earned from 1 July 1993 to 30 June 1994

1995/96 profits earned in the year ended 30 June 1994.

Accordingly, the opening year forms the basis of between two and three years' assessments to establish the practice on the preceding year basis. However, if the profits actually earned in the second and third years of assessment are lower than the profits which would be taxed according to these rules, the practice can elect to be taxed on the actual profits earned in those two years.

Taxing a partnership at its cessation

When the partnership ends, there will be profits covering a period of between one and two years which do not form the basis of any assessment.

The assessment for the final period from 6 April to the date of cessation is based upon actual profits earned during that period. The assessments for the two immediately previous years may, at the discretion of the Inland Revenue, be increased to the actual profits of those two years.

For example, if a practice ceased on 30 June 1993, the assessment would be:

1990/91 year ended 30 June 1989

1991/92 year ended 30 June 1990 or increased to profits earned from 6 April 1991 to 5 April 1992.

Proposed changes to the taxation of the self-employed

The Government plans to implement proposals for simplifying the taxation of the self-employed. The provisions set out below are based on the Finance Bill which was published on 11 January 1994 prior to any amendments which may arise before the new legislation is finally incorporated in the Finance Act 1994.

It is proposed to:

- abolish the complex preceding year basis of assessment for the self-employed
- abolish partners' joint and several liability for partnership tax
- allow taxpayers who complete a tax return to choose between assessing themselves and working out how much tax is due on their total income (in which case they would have to submit their tax return by 31 January following the end of the tax year), or allowing the Inland Revenue to make the assessment (in which case the tax return would have to be submitted by 1 October following the end of the tax year)
- abolish the 'schedular' system, thus bringing together all the taxpayer's income from all sources on one tax statement, with one tax bill.

The new rules relating to self-assessment and the abolition of the 'schedular' system are expected to take effect from the tax year 1996/97.

Abolishing the preceding year basis

The preceding year basis of assessment would be replaced by a current year basis, so that the accounting period ending in the tax year will form the basis of assessment for that year.

It had been suggested in an earlier consultative document that fiscal accounting should be compulsory, ie all self-employed individuals would have to draw up their accounts to 5 April. This has been dropped and the self-employed will continue to choose their own accounting year end.

Indeed, under the current year basis of assessment the choice of an optimum accounting date will continue to be important. For example, liability for the first full year of the new system (1997/98) would be based on the accounting period ending in the year 5 April 1998. This could be either the year ending 31 March 1998 or the year ending 30 April 1997. Therefore, it is still possible to defer the payment of tax on profits by choosing the optimum accounting date. (*See* Figures 6.4 and 6.5.)

PARTNERSHIP TAXATION 71

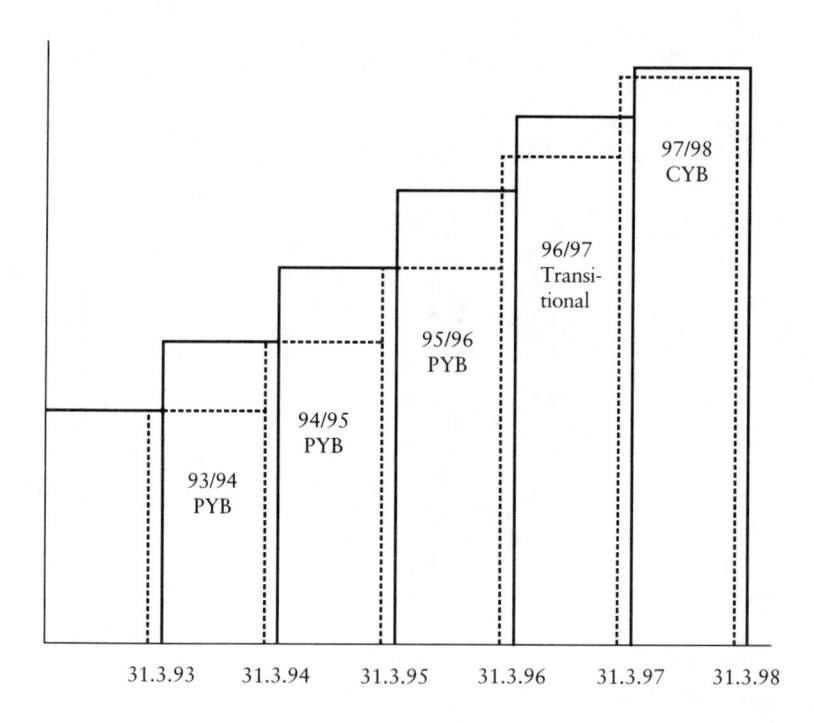

Figure 6.4 Introduction of current year basis (CYB) for accounting year end 31 March

Under the current year basis, it is proposed that tax will still be payable, in two equal instalments on 31 January in the tax year and 31 July following the end of the tax year. Each instalment will be based on one half of the actual tax liability for the previous year, with any balance of outstanding tax due for the current year payable on the following 31 January. Therefore, for the tax year 1997/98, the two interim instalments would be payable on 31 January 1998 and 31 July 1998, with any balance due payable on 31 January 1999. This still applies if your year end is 30 June 1997 or 31 March 1998.

Tax returns

Partners will have to submit personal tax returns by 31 January following the end of the tax year which will include his or her share of the partnership profit assessable in that tax year. The return will also have to include

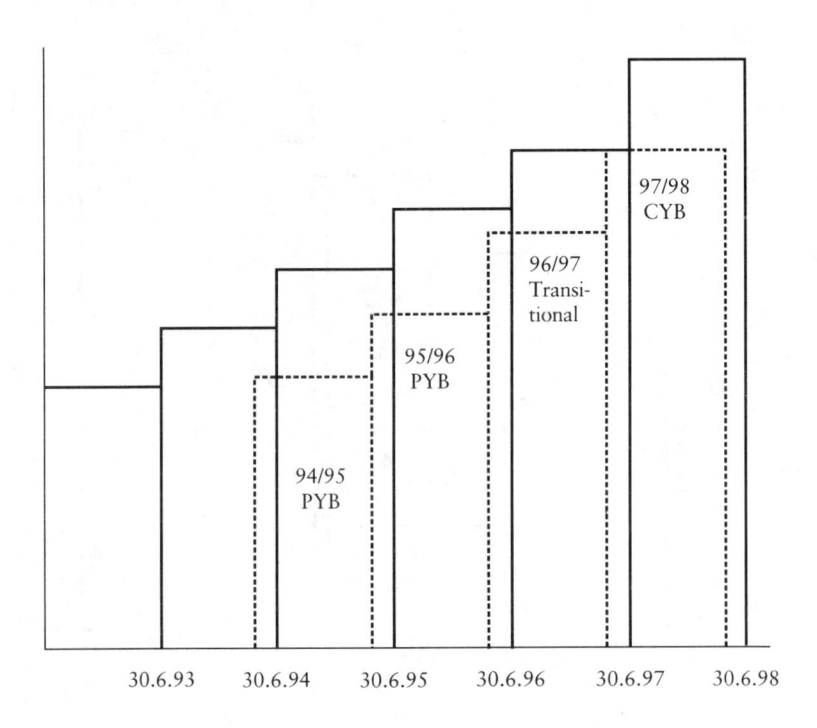

Figure 6.5 Introduction of the current year basis of assessment (CYB) for accounting year end 30 June

the calculation of the income tax and any capital gains tax liability. If the taxpayer prefers that the Inland Revenue calculate the tax payable, the Return would have to be submitted by 30 September following the end of the tax year.

Partnerships will also have to file a separate partnership return which will have the same filing date of 31 January following the end of the tax year. For example, a partnership would have to submit its return for 1997/98 by 1 January 1999 which would incorporate the profits based on its accounting period ending in the year ended 5 April 1998 which could therefore be the year ended 31 March 1998 or the year ended 30 June 1997. The Return will have to be submitted by a nominated partner and will include a list of partners, their private addresses and tax references. It will also include a partnership statement showing the trading profit or loss, together with bank interest and any other sources of income, and also capital gains and charges on income, and the allocation of these profits between the partners.

Penalties

There will be a system of penalties to encourage people to submit returns on time and to pay their tax by the due dates. There will be three types of penalties:

- surcharges for the late payment of tax
- penalties for the late submission of returns, and
- other penalties.

Surcharges for the late payment of tax

These will not apply to the two interim payments, but if the tax paid by 31 January following the year of assessment is less than the tax due, the surcharge will be:

• tax paid up to 28 days of the due date, ie normally by 28 February	Nil
• tax paid between 28 days and six months of the due date	5% of that tax
• tax paid more than six months after the due date	10% of that tax.

Interest is payable in addition to the surcharge and, surcharges themselves will carry interest. The Inland Revenue will have the right to mitigate such surcharges if they see fit.

Penalties for the late submission of returns

The penalty for the failure to submit a Return will be £100 plus up to £60 a day for any failure continuing after the Commissioners have directed a Return to be submitted.

If the Return is submitted more than six months late, the penalty is £200 instead of £100 and if more than 12 months late there will be a tax related penalty of 100% of the tax. These penalties apply to both personal and partnership tax returns.

Other penalties

There will also be a penalty of up to 10% of the tax for incorrect returns. In the case of a partnership return each partner is liable for the penalty in respect of his share of the profits.

Interest

Interest will apply to interim payments as well as final payments and run from the due date of the payment.

The choice of a favourable accounting date can defer submission of the accounts and computations, and payment of the final tax liability, by between 10 and 21 months after the end of the accounting year. Given the application of interest and penalties set out above it could be advantageous to avoid unnecessarily tight deadlines.

However, in choosing the most appropriate accounting year end, consideration must also be given to the tax position of retiring partners which is considered later in this chapter.

The transitional year

It is proposed that 1996/97 will be a transitional year. To move smoothly from the preceding year basis system of tax to the current year basis, 1996/97 will be taxed on the profit for 12 months out of the period between the basis periods for 1995/96 and 1997/98. This will generally be one half of the profits for the two year period ending in 1996/97.

Accordingly, with a 30 June year end, 1996/97 will be taxed on one half of the profits for the year ended 30 June 1995 and the year ended 30 June 1996. This means that, effectively, the equivalent of one year's profits will not be taxed.

Although this is an attractive idea, it must be remembered that one year's expenses will not be allowed against income tax. It is therefore important to review the timing of expenditure and where possible bring expenditure forward to before the commencment of the first accounting period which will be assessable in 1996/97, eg with a June year end, incur expenditure before 30 June 1994 or defer it until after the end of the second relevant accounting period, eg after 30 June 1996. This would apply particularly to repairs and renewals and redecorations where some flexibility in the timing of the expenditure may be available.

It is also worth considering buying rather than leasing assets, as capital allowances will not be affected by the 24 month averaging rule. Full relief will, therefore, be available via the capital allowance system, whereas tax relief will only be available on half the lease cost in that two year period.

If the practice makes pension contributions for its staff, contributions can be paid before the end of the year, which forms the basis for 1995/96, so as to minimize any contribution paid in the period assessable in 1996/97.

In these circumstances, it may also be worthwhile reviewing a partnership's capital funding to determine whether it is advantageous for a partnership loan to be replaced by individual bank loans for the purpose of funding the partnership's capital. Tax relief would then be obtained individually on an actual year basis through the individual partners' personal tax returns. This is usually advantageous in any circumstances because it accelerates the tax relief. However, it would be particularly beneficial as some of the relief will otherwise be lost.

Partnership changes

The concept of joint and several liability to tax on a partnership assessment will no longer apply. Instead a partner's share of partnership profits will be treated as a separate trade carried out by the partner. Therefore, a partner joining or leaving the practice will have no effect on the other continuing partners.

An incoming partner will be treated as if he had set up a new business when he joins the partnership and hence the opening year rules will apply to that partner. An outgoing partner will be treated as if his business had ceased and therefore the cessation rules will apply to his share of profit and overlap relief will be available to offset against that final assessable profit. These special rules are set out below.

Starting and ending partnerships

It had originally been announced that no special rules would be required for partnership commencements and cessations.

These special rules, as operated under the existing preceding year basis system caused the main mismatch between profit earned and profits taxed and make it difficult for most taxpayers to understand how the system works.

Under the proposals in the Finance Bill, the broad principle remains that over the lifetime of a business all profits earned will be taxed once and only once.

However, there are now some proposals for special rules to apply to the opening and closing years of a business, and also where there is a change of accounting date, resulting in there not being a 12 month period ending in the year of assessment.

Opening year rules

The following basis periods will apply to new businesses and to a new partner joining the practice.

Year 1: Actual profit from commencement to 5 April

Year 2: either,
    (a) 12 months ending with the accounting date in the year, or
    (b) 12 months from commencment date, if there is no such 12 month period

Year 3: 12 months ending with the accounting date.

For example, the following basis periods would apply if a practice commenced on 1 July 1998 and alternatively made up its accounts to:

(i)   30 June 1999, or
(ii) 30 April 2000, or
(iii) 31 March 2000.

		(i)	(ii)	(iii)
Year 1	1998/99	9 months to 5.4.99	9 months to 5.4.99	9 months to 5.4.99
Year 2	1999/00	12 months to 30.6.99 (a)	12 months to 30.6.99 (b)	12 months to 31.3.00 (a)
Year 3	2000/01	12 months to 30.6.00	12 months to 30.4.00	12 months to 31.3.01

Taking the example in (i) above, the profits from 1 July 1998 to 5 April 1999 will be taxed twice, once in 1998/99 and again in 1999/2000. This period is therefore treated as an overlap and overlap relief will be available on these profits as explained later.

Closing year rules

When a practice ceases, the profits to be taken into account for the last year will be those arising from the end of the basis period in the preceding year.

For example, if a practice which made up its accounts to 30 June each year ceases on 30 June 2000 the assessable profits would be:

1999/2000   year to 30 June 1999
2000/2001   12 months from 1 July 1999 to 30 June 2000.

However, if instead of ceasing on 30 June 2000 it made up its final accounts to 31 March 2001, the position would then be:

1999/2000   year to 30 June 1999
2000/2001   21 months from 1 July 1999 to 31 March 2001.

Accordingly, in the first and last year of a business, a period other than 12 months can fall to be taxed.

These closing year rules will apply to individual partners when they retire from the practice.

It will be seen that under the new system a partner retiring on 30 June 2000 will pay tax on the whole of the 2000/2001 assessment even though he has retired just three months into that tax year.

This additional nine months' liability will however be reduced by overlap relief which in the case of a 30 June year end will generally be $9/_{12}$ths of the 1997/98 assessable profits. *See* later.

If, instead of drawing accounts up to 30 June, a practice draws its accounts up to 31 March, then a partner would not suffer any charge to tax after the date of retirement from the practice. For example, a practice made up its accounts to 31 March 2000 and a partner retires on that date, his final assessable profit would be: 1999/2000 year to 31 March 2000.

However, if the practice had made up its accounts to 31 March 1997/98 then there would be no overlap relief arising from that period, as the assessable profits would have been based on the year ended 31 March 1998.

Overlap relief

As referred to above, the Finance Bill has introduced a new form of relief called overlap relief which will apply where profits are taxed more than once. However, the relief will only be given on the earlier of:

- a change in the accounting date which results in an assessment based on a period of more than 12 months, or
- the cessation of the trade. This applies to a partner leaving a practice but in that case would affect only the outgoing partner.

For businesses commencing before 6 April 1994, 1996/97 is the transitional year between the two tax systems and 1997/98 is the first full year of the new system. Taking the example of a partner whose share of the profits in the year ended 30 June 1997 is £60,000 the assessment would be:

1997/98   01.07.96 to 30.06.97   <u>£60,000</u>

The period 1 July 1996 to 5 April 1997 is treated as an overlap period. Overlap relief of £45,000 will be available either when the whole practice ceases, or on that partner's retirement, or in a year for which the basis period is longer than 12 months, ie if there is a change of accounting date.

This relief will therefore be available to most partners as a Case II deduction when they retire in their final year of assessment. This is intended to compensate them for the fact that under the new current year system, if a partner were to retire on say 30 June 1998, then he would share in the full 1998/99 assessment rather than in just $3/_{12}$ths of that assessment as he would do under the present system. The overlap relief is accordingly offset against that final assessment in order to reduce that liability.

Capital allowances and personal expenses

The treatment for the relief of capital allowances is to change to that currently used for companies. Capital allowances will accordingly be treated as a deduction in computing trading profits in the same way as expenses are treated. The relief for capital allowances will therefore be tied to the accounting period rather than the year of assessment.

Relief for all the partners' personal capital allowances and personal expense claims will also be given in the same way and these will have to be included on the partnership tax return as a deduction from the accounts profit for relief to be claimed.

New businesses commencing after 5 April 1994

In the case of a new practice starting up after 5 April 1994 the new current year basis will apply immediately. Therefore, the opening year rules set out earlier will apply, and also partners would be subject to individual assessment on their share of the practice profits. This position also applies to partnerships deemed to have commenced following a cessation for tax purposes after 5 April 1994.

The application of these opening year rules could present a practical problem for partners joining a practice before 5 April in a tax year where the accounts are drawn up to a date late in the calendar year. For example, a partner joining a practice on 1 February 1999 where the partnership accounts are made up to 31 December 1999 would have to include on his tax return for the year 1998/99 his share of the profits for the period from 1 February to 5 April 1999. This return must be submitted by 31 January 2000, although it is very unlikely the partnership accounts for the year ended 31 December 1999 could be finalized by then.

On any partnership changes occurring between 6 April 1994 and 6 April 1997 it will be necessary to consider if it may be beneficial for the partners to treat that change as a cessation for tax purposes in order to opt into the new system prematurely.

Cessations before 6 April 1997

Any practice which ceases before 6 April 1997 will be assessed on the existing rules.

Cessation between 6 April 1997 and 5 April 1999

Any business which has been subject to the transitional arrangements in 1996/97 and then ceases prior to 5 April 1998 may be assessed on revised figures for 1995/96 and 1996/97. Effectively the Inland Revenue have the option of applying the existing closing year rules which apply under the preceding year basis whereby the assessments may be revised to actual basis. If a business ceases between 6 April 1998 and 5 April 1999 the Inland Revenue have the right to adjust just 1996/97 to actual.

7 Exploitation in Partnerships

Chris Hughes

Introduction

Many partnership agreements reflect a disparity in bargaining power between the partners. This may take various forms, including very unequal profit shares, an unfair allocation of existing and new patients, onerous conditions and working arrangements selectively imposed on some but not all partners, a lack of influence over the running of the partnership, and restrictive covenants which are either excessive or imposed on some but not all partners. In some cases, a partner may either never reach parity or remain on a fixed salary instead of receiving a profit share.

Such inequalities cause problems for both the partnership as a whole and its individual partners. In particular, they raise a crucial question: how unequal can a partnership be before it ceases to be a partnership? If, in reality, a partnership cannot be said to exist, the financial implications of this position for the partners can be serious.

Even if a partnership actually exists, many of the more onerous terms of agreement referred to above can be problematic; eg penalty clauses, restrictive practices and sexually discriminatory provisions are often unenforceable.

This chapter looks at some legal consequences of inequality and exploitation in partnerships and explains where there is some protection for exploited partners.

Who cares if a partnership is genuine?

In relation to medical partnerships, it is necessary to consider who is affected by whether or not a partnership between the practitioners truly exists. Generally speaking, patients are not affected; the practice continues to provide a service and the GPs are covered by their medical defence organization membership. Similarly, a tradesman dealing with a partnership in good faith can still bring proceedings in respect of a contract entered into by an ostensible partner. The employees of the partnership are also unlikely to be affected.

Apart from the partners themselves, those persons most directly concerned with this aspect of the partnership are the Inland Revenue and the FHSA. There are substantial tax advantages to be gained from working in partnership as opposed to working as an employee, not least in relation to the treatment of expenses and being taxed on a preceding year basis. Many payments made by the FHSA are only payable to a principal, in particular the various practice allowances which added together can amount to a substantial sum. The FHSA is required to ensure that it only pays out money in accordance with the NHS General Medical Services (GMS) regulations, which define the circumstances in which a medical practitioner is eligible to receive payments as a principal.

Criteria for determining whether a partnership exists

The question as to whether a partnership exists is determined by matters of both fact and law. It is necessary to look at the question in the round because no single factor is necessarily decisive. In addition to any written agreement, the intentions of the parties can be inferred from their words and actions, which may serve to qualify any written agreement.

The statutory definition of a partnership is 'the relationship which exists between persons carrying on a business in common with a view to profit'. There is no exhaustive definition of a partnership, although there is some guidance in the Partnership Act 1890 (see Box 7.1), and the NHS GMS regulations indicate when a FHSA regards someone as a partner (see Box 7.2).

The phrase 'share in the profits', as used in the GMS regulations, implies that an FHSA will be concerned if it knows of circumstances where a partner is not being rewarded for his or her efforts by a profit share, but is being paid instead a fixed salary unrelated to the practice's actual profits. The FHSA may conclude that such an arrangement does not constitute a partnership, and if so, it may be obliged to remove patients from the list of the so-called partnership. In addition to list size problems, FHSAs may be obliged to investigate whether the practice has been overpaid in circumstances where there are doubts about the genuineness of a partnership.

> **Box 7.1: The Partnership Act 1890 – rules for determining whether a partnership exists**
>
> 1 Joint ownership of property, whether the owners share the profits made from the use of the property or not, or the sharing of gross returns of a business whether or not the people sharing the returns jointly own property used in the business, do not in themselves create a partnership.
>
> 2 The receipt of a share in profits of a business is prima facie evidence that he or she is a partner, but the receipt of such a share or of a payment varying with the profits of a business does not in itself make him or her a partner.
>
> [Extract from Section 2 of the Partnership Act 1890]

> **Box 7.2: GMS regulation 24(4)**
>
> For a doctor to be treated as a partner, the FHSA must be satisfied that he or she:
>
> 1 discharges the duties and exercises the powers of a principal in connection with the practice of the partnership
>
> 2 is available for a minimum number of hours and receives a minimum share of profits relating to the hours worked, at three levels*:
>
> - approved hours of not less than 26 per week and receives profits amounting to not less than one third of the share of the partner with the greatest share (full-time or job-share); or
> - less than 26 approved hours but not less than 19 per week, and receives not less than one quarter of the profit share of the partner with the greatest share (part-time practitioner); or
> - less than 19 approved hours but not less than 13 hours per week, and receives not less than one fifth of the profit share of the partner with the greatest share (half-time practitioner).

See also page 103.

Such an investigation can be extremely stressful to the GPs concerned; it requires them to present highly detailed evidence and may be financially damaging.

How one FHSA judged that a partnership was genuine

An FHSA investigated a partnership following an allegation that one partner was in fact an employee. Several years' allowances were at stake. The FHSA Medical Services Committee made the following findings.

- The doctors had notified the FHSA that they were all principals and none received a share less than a third of any principal.
- The accountant confirmed that no partner received a lesser share than a third of any principal.
- All the partners had signed a partnership restriction clause.
- The junior partner had recently been offered an increased share in the partnership.
- The bank confirmed that two out of three partners were cheque signatories and all were liable on the account.
- All three doctors appeared on practice documents.
- All three doctors' signatures appeared on applications relating to the use of the deputizing service.
- In all correspondence with the FHSA, the doctors had stated that they were partners.

The Medical Service Committee, after considering the facts, concluded that there was a partnership and no sums were due to be repaid.

Figure 7.1 A case study from the BMA files

FHSA seeks substantial repayment after partnership found to be bogus

A complaint was received from a junior partner in the practice that he was not fairly treated and was not in fact a partner. The FHSA Medical Services Committee investigated and made the following findings.

- The junior partner was paid a salary, not a share of the profits.
- The junior partner was taxed on Schedule E, not Schedule D.
- The partnership restriction clause only restricted the activities of the junior partner.

- The junior partner was not a signatory on cheques.
- The junior partner took no part in the management of practice.
- The junior partner's list was far smaller than that of the senior partners, despite a considerable length of service in the partnership.

The Medical Service Committee considered these facts, concluded that there was no partnership between the junior and other partners, and advised the FHSA to seek repayment of several tens of thousands of pounds worth of practice allowances.

Figure 7.2   A case study from the BMA files

Over many years, the courts have examined contracts to determine whether a real partnership exists:

'Two parties enter into a transaction and say "It is hereby declared and agreed that there is no partnership between us". The Court pays no regard to that. The Court looks at the transaction and says, "Is this, in point of law, really a partnership?" It is not in the least conclusive that the parties have used a term or language intended to indicate that the transaction is not that which in law it is.'[1]

Almost as a matter of course persons who share profits and losses will be partners, but this does not mean that, even if they are partners, they will all be entitled to manage or dissolve the firm.

Salaried partners

A similar problem of definition arises with salaried partners. A salaried partner is usually someone who is effectively an employee, but who is held by the outside world to be a partner; remuneration is usually by salary or sometimes by a profit share. The difficulty is that a 'salaried partner' is denied the normal rights and duties of a partnership, ie he or she does not contribute to capital, share in the profits and losses (normally), or participate in managing the practice. In a leading case,[2] the Judge, analysing the position of a salaried partner, concluded:

'It seems to me impossible to say that, as a matter of law, a salaried partner is or is not necessarily a partner in the true sense. He may or may not be a partner, depending on the facts. What must be done is to look at the substance of the relationship between the parties.

> If there is a plain contract of [employer] and [employee], and the only qualification of that relationship is that the employee is being held out as a partner, the name 'salaried partner' seems perfectly apt for him; and yet he will be no partner in relation to other members of the firm. At the other extreme, there may be a full partnership deed under which all the partners save one take a share of the profits, with that one being paid a fixed salary not dependent on profits; yet I do not see why he should not be a true partner, at all events if he is entitled to a share in the profits on a winding-up . . . If I am right in this, then it seems to me that one must in every case look at the terms of the relationship to ascertain whether or not it creates a true partnership.'

If court or an FHSA is trying to determine whether a partnership exists, it will consider a wide range of evidence relating to how the business is actually being run. It is not possible to provide an exhaustive list of all those factors it will wish to take into account, but the following are some which have been held to be relevant:

- no participation in management
- no right to see accounts
- no share of profits
- no access to cheque book
- no power to sign cheques
- salary permanently fixed significantly below a partner's share
- deduction of tax and national insurance
- onerous conditions imposed, which do not apply to other partners.

If GPs claim they are partners when they are not, they may incur not only a civil liability to repay any allowances incorrectly paid to the practice, but they could also be criminally liable. This is because the Inland Revenue and FHSAs, having dealt with a partnership on the presumption that it is a true partnership – ie allowing concessions and authorizing payments – will not hesitate in initiating legal proceedings if they discover that the partnership is not a genuine one.

Penalty clauses

One option which some practices have very occasionally considered is to impose penalty clauses in partnership agreements. This could take the form of a clause in which each partner agrees to pay a certain sum in case of the infringement by that partner of any agreement contained in the provisions of the partnership contract. Such a clause may apply to all partners or only to incoming partners. However, clauses of this nature may not be enforceable. The basic rule is that, if the sum specified in the clause is a reasonable attempt to estimate the likely loss which the breach would cause, then it is an enforceable provision in the agreement. If, however, the sum specified bears no real relationship to any such loss, then it is not likely to be an enforceable provision. The courts have clearly laid down that how such a payment is described does not matter and the question of whether the clauses are actually enforceable has to be decided in the light of the circumstances at the time the agreement was made, not at the time the breach occurred.

Penalty clauses of damage are generally not worth including in partnership agreements. Those matters which might be covered by these clauses are generally better dealt with on a 'knock for knock' basis, eg if a partner at short notice has to ask one of his colleagues to cover the surgery, should he really be required to pay some money over? If he should, then it is likely that the sum of £50 would be a fairer assessment of damages and enforceable, whereas £500 would be unreasonable and would therefore be unenforceable as a penalty clause.

Sex discrimination

The European Community (EC) has legislated for equal treatment between self-employed men and women. This implies the absence of all discrimination on the grounds of sex, marital or family status. UK legislation implements this (at least in part) and provides that it is unlawful to discriminate in partnerships. However, the UK law on sex discrimination is in a state of flux and uncertainty; it is not clear how far EC law has been properly implemented, or what is the precise content of EC rights. Yet it is clear that any discrimination in offering a partnership, and in its terms, is unlawful.

> **Box 7.3: Common areas of discrimination in partnership agreements**
>
> - Maternity provisions less favourable than sickness arrangements.
> - Longer time to reach parity.
> - No entitlement for time off for ante-natal care.
> - Unreasonable requirement for an early return to work.

Restrictive covenants

Restrictive covenants are generally considered not to be in the public interest. However, they may be permissible if their terms are no wider than is strictly necessary. Courts take a less favourable view of restrictive covenants between an employer and employee than between persons, such as partners, who work together on a more equal footing. Two key questions need to be addressed.

1 Is it reasonable in terms of the public interest? There are no clear cut cases where a covenant which has been upheld as being reasonable in the interests of the parties, has been deemed to be against the public interest. Although it has been established that medical goodwill can in principle be protected by a restrictive covenant, this is unlikely to provide sufficient grounds in itself to justify a covenant.

2 Is it reasonable in the interests of the parties? Is there a legitimate interest capable of protection, which is not excessive in respect of the geographical area covered, its duration or the activities which are prohibited?

Area covered by a restrictive covenant

The area covered by a so-called 'brass plate' restriction should be no greater than is needed to protect the business. Since NHS GPs work in defined practice areas, it is reasonable to assume that a covenant not to practise should be based on these areas. If an area clause is part of a restrictive covenant, its range must be decided in the light of the practice's social and geographical environment. An agreement not to practise within two miles of the premises has a quite different impact in a rural setting than in an urban setting. To illustrate, in a significant case[3] involving an employment agency, a restrictive covenant which prevented a former employee from running an agency within a comparatively narrow geographical area was judged to be too wide, and therefore unreasonable, because it covered most of the City of London. Thus, any area restriction must be carefully tailored to reflect the needs of the practice, if it is to be enforceable.

In addition, or as an alternative to a 'brass plate' restriction, a non-solicitation clause may be used. This prevents an outgoing partner from offering services to former patients of the practice for a restricted period of time. Such a restriction is less likely to be held as unreasonable because it only applies to existing patients and does not restrict dealings with persons who are not patients. However, its breach may be harder to prove than a breach of a 'brass plate' restriction.

Duration of restrictive covenants

There are no reported cases where an otherwise reasonable restriction in an agreement between GPs was dismissed by the courts solely because of its duration. However, a 10 year restriction was judged to be 'impossible, in any circumstances, to support at trial'.[4] In another case,[5] two years was deemed to be quite reasonable.

Prohibited activities

In one case,[6] it was held that the term 'medical practitioner' was too broad because it prohibited hospital practice. If the scope of a clause goes beyond the actual or reasonably anticipated activities of the practice at the time of the agreement, it is liable to be considered unenforceable.

Mutuality

Another key issue which affects reasonableness is mutuality. In a case relating to solicitors,[7] the observation was made:

> 'On this question, the mutuality of the contract is a most important consideration. The contract applied equally to all the partners. None of them could tell whether he might find himself in a position of being a retiring partner subject to the restriction in clause 28, or a continuing partner with an interest to enforce the restriction. It was at least as favourable to the defendant as to the more senior partners.'

In other words, any restrictive covenant has to apply equally to all partners.

Although courts will not normally allow opinions of reasonableness as evidence, they will take account of custom and practice within a profession. If the covenant is wider than is customary, then there is a greater risk of it being found invalid. In this respect, the Medical Practices Committee's guidance, which suggests that a restriction not to engage in NHS general medical practice for a period of two years within a radius of two miles is an acceptable maximum, may be viewed by courts as evidence of a customary arrangement within general practice.

General points relating to covenants

The following points should be noted.

- On a general dissolution of the partnership, the restraint will fall.
- (a) If an outgoing partner cannot be persuaded to resign from the local FHSA medical list, it is likely that he or she will be able to continue to practise from new premises, unless the court grants an injunction to enforce the covenant. If a partnership continues as a 'partnership at will', the restraint will normally fall;[8] but

    (b) In a case referred to previously,[5] the court seemed to consider that patients were 'patients of the practice' rather than of individual GPs; a view not easily reconciled with the NHS GMS regulations, but commonly held.
- A salaried partner is likely to be treated as an employee for the purposes of deciding whether a covenant is reasonable. Taking into account his or her normal right to practise medicine freely, it will be easier for him or her to show that the restriction is unreasonable.

Goodwill

The standing of a practice in its community is important and valuable to its partners. Although they may wish to protect their goodwill by means of a restrictive covenant, the statutory prohibition laid down by the NHS Act 1977 means they may not in any way buy or sell goodwill. The Medical Practices Committee (MPC) is responsible for policing the prohibition and may, if requested, certify that any proposed transaction does not breach this ban. Schedule 10 of the Act gives details of matters which will be regarded as a sale of goodwill (*see* Box 7.4); any breach of these may incur criminal liability.

> **Box 7.4: Statutory guidance on unlawful sales of medical goodwill**
>
> The following arrangements are unlawful.
>
> - A GP selling or letting his or her practice premises to another GP, for use as practice premises, for substantially more than they would be worth if they had not been used by a GP.
> - A partnership agreement where a new partner gives valuable consideration (other than working in the business) for joining the partnership.
> - A partnership agreement where a partner is paid to retire.
> - A partnership agreement where a partner works for substantially less than his or her services are worth.

The MPC has also referred to other matters which it considers to be evidence of a sale of goodwill. These include a failure to reach parity within three years, unfair allocation of profit and workload, and restrictive covenants which are over-restrictive and not mutual. Many of those matters which cast doubt whether a partnership exists (*see* pages 82–86) are relevant when deciding whether there has been a sale of goodwill.

Conclusion

It is clear that, if a partnership agreement is substantially unbalanced and unfair to one party, then it is likely that the partnership will not be a stable and successful relationship. This is because it is not based on a level of mutual trust which is essential to any long-term partnership.

Many of the contractual terms which introduce unfairness into partnership agreements also pose practical difficulties. The extent of these may be such as to lead a court to conclude that there is no partnership; thus any payments previously received from the FHSA, which are contingent on the partner being a principal, may have to be repaid. In any event, penalty clauses and restrictive covenants may be unenforceable.

An incoming partner faced with an agreement with such terms should think long and hard before joining the practice. Although there is a temptation to join and hope that things will resolve themselves in due course, there is the danger that they will not. The new partner may find himself or herself in an impossible position after a few years, with no rights in the partnership, a small list and no ability to improve his or her position without moving on.

[1] Weiner v Harris [1910] 1 K.B. 285

[2] Stekel v Ellice [1973] 1 All E.R. 465

[3] Office Angels Ltd v Rainer-Thomas [1991] I.R.L.R. 214 CA

[4] Pandit v Shah (unrep.) Lindley and Banks on Partnership (16 Ed.) 1990 Sweet & Maxwell, London

[5] Kerr v Morris [1986] 3 All E.R. 217

[6] Routh v Jones [1947] 1 All E.R. 758

[7] Deacon v Bridge [1984] A.C. 705

[8] Hensman v Traill [1980] 124 S.J. 776

8 Sharing Workload and Profits

Lorna Dunlop

Introduction

The relationship between profit shares and workload lies at the heart of the partnership and can be a major source of conflict. Each partner's share should reflect his or her contribution to the work of the practice. This is not just because there should be a common desire to ensure that partners neither exploit nor deceive one another, but also because an equitable business relationship is an essential precondition for the collegiate relationships which should permeate general practice. The process of quantifying and formalizing the workload-profit equation can in itself reassure partners that there is a genuine commitment to establishing an equitable relationship.

This chapter discusses those factors to be taken into account when relating workload and profit, and outlines how a points system can formalize intuitive attempts to assess workload, enabling those assumptions which are often implicit in partnership arrangements to be made more explicit. The points scored for various activities need to be reviewed regularly to ensure that they correspond to actual work being done and incorporate any necessary amendments. The scores also need to be revised whenever a significant change in the partnership occurs, such as the appointment or retirement of a partner.

Measuring workload

In order to measure the distribution of workload among partners, its components need to be identified and analysed, including, for example:

- number of home visits over, say, a three month period
- number of surgery consultations (classified according to whether they are emergency cases, new non-urgent cases, return attendances

initiated by the patient, or return attendances intiated by the doctor) analysed over, say, 10 consecutive surgery sessions
- patient waiting times for routine appointments, analysed by each partner
- weekly pattern of each partner's work, eg number of routine surgery appointments, minor surgery sessions, child health clinics, diabetic or asthmatic clinics, maternity clinics.

If both the qualitative and quantitative aspects of workload are measured as precisely as possible, a partnership should be able to assess how it is distributed. This exercise can also indicate how working arrangements (or partnership shares) could be more equitable. Although a detailed analysis of this kind may be seen as putting at risk the stability of a partnership, it does provide a 'snapshot' which can reassure partners that a serious effort is being made to ensure that partnership arrangements are equitable. It can also act as a catalyst for change – the data generated can resolve specific partnership problems such as:

- the workload implications of an unequal distribution among partners of return consultations or 'non-attenders', which may in turn influence the distribution of new presentations
- an unequal distribution among partners of different types of clinical cases.

Parity

An incoming partner usually receives a significantly smaller share of profits on joining the partnership than that received by established partners. The actual size of this reduced share should take account of the new partner's previous experience and the time required to become familiar with the practice and its patients, and should be justifiable according to these factors. Inevitably, however, market forces also affect both the level of the initial share and the time taken to reach parity.

The minimum profit shares specified in the NHS GMS regulations are a useful starting point from which to calculate a new partner's share, although they may be too low if the new partner assumes a full-time commitment. The partnership deed should specify how a new partner's profit share will be increased and the length of time that will be taken to reach parity. It is still generally held that parity should be achieved within three years of becoming a partner.

Out-of-hours commitment

A practice's profit sharing ratios should reflect the workload implications of its out-of-hours arrangements. Unless a practice has subcontracted all of its out-of-hours care to a deputizing service, it has to decide how individual partners should be compensated for this work in terms of their partnership shares.

In a small partnership, out-of-hours work can be a comparatively large proportion of total workload, and therefore it is likely to have a more significant influence on profit sharing ratios than in larger practices. In the latter, it may comprise a smaller proportion of total workload in terms of time commitment, although the actual amount of work done by the duty doctor is far greater.

Partners can be compensated in various ways for out-of-hours work. Whichever method is adopted, it should be based on an agreement between the partners that profit sharing ratios take account of each partner's on-call commitment. This general approach can accommodate a variety of ways of organizing and remunerating out-of-hours care, including the following.

- The practice pays a retainer to a deputizing service, allowing each partner to choose when and whether to use it and to pay any consequential charges.

- The practice pays each partner fees for on-call work, or forms a limited company to employ partners as locums to cover this work.

- On-call work is divided equally between partners, who also divide their income equally.

Relating workload and profit

The partnership deed should specify how each partner's profit share is calculated, and the timing and size of any future increases (eg the staged increases required to reach parity). The agreement should also distinguish between partnership income (included in profit shares) and personal income, classifying as practice or personal income each of the following income sources:

- hospital work
- occupational health work
- night visit fees

- PGEA
- commissioning and fundholding
- prizes, legacies and awards
- seniority payments
- fees for lectures or writing
- private practice (including public sector insurance certification).

There are many different ways of allocating income from these activities; ranging from dividing all of it strictly according to partnership shares, to allowing each partner to retain the income he or she earns. No system is perfect and each practice should devise a system for its own use which it believes to be equitable. A possible 'compromise' solution is the points system described below.

The points system

The scoring system described below offers a comprehensive and systematic method of measuring workload. The point scoring system may be regarded as 'fixed' or 'flexible', depending on the time-span elapsing between reviews. Under a fixed system, profit shares are more or less stable until and unless significant changes require a review. Under a flexible points system, profit shares could change as frequently as monthly if changes in workload justify this.

The following description of how to calculate and allocate points applies to a fixed points system, although its methodology is equally relevant to a flexible points system. At first sight, the whole system may appear daunting, complex and too formal. However, it does provide a starting point for practices which wish to improve their approach to the measurement of workload. It contains the key elements most practices need to address and can serve as a checklist to ensure that none are neglected. Above all, a point scoring system helps to objectify the measurement of workload and profit: partners usually find it easier to discuss relativities between weightings and scores than the size of individual shares and profits.

Calculating points

Each partner should allocate his or her work among an agreed list of units of medical time (eg morning, afternoon and evening surgeries; Saturday morning surgeries; on call – weekday nights and weekends) and if a

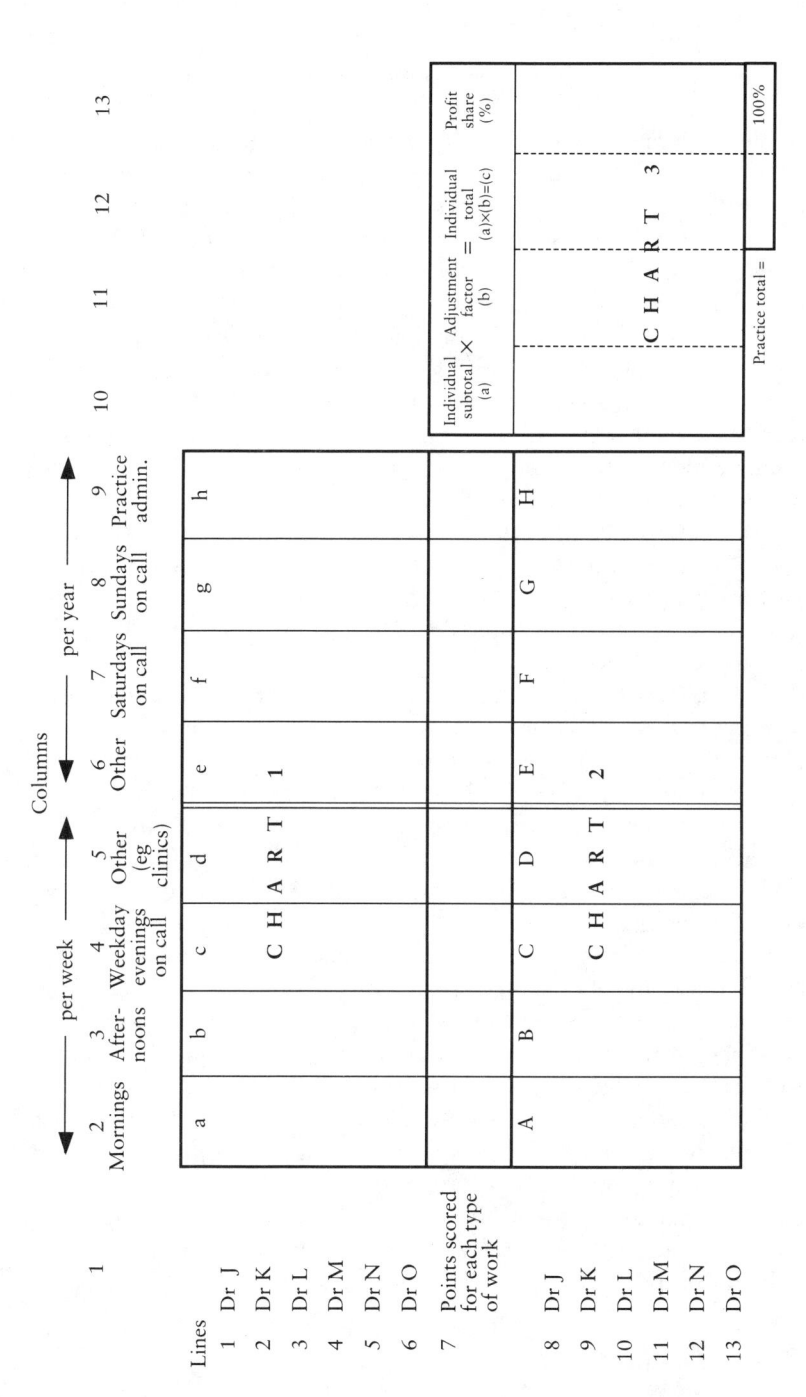

Figure 8.1 Sharing workload and profits: the points system

practice considers it necessary, even more specific divisions within units should be agreed.

The charts in Figure 8.1 should be completed. There should be a horizontal list of heads covering each category (and, where appropriate, sub-category) of units of medical time, which the partnership has agreed to use to allocate its work for the purpose of measuring both quantitative and qualitative aspects of workload. Columns 2–5 are for normal weekly commitments and columns 6–9 for less frequent commitments, which should be calculated on an annual basis. For example, if Dr J normally works one Sunday in six on-call, the number 9 should be entered in column 8, line 1 (ie g = 9). Column 1, spanning charts 1 and 2, simply lists all partners.

Chart 1 shows the amount of work done by each partner in respect of each unit of medical time, on both a weekly and annual basis.

The key to this scoring system is agreement among partners on the value to be attached to each type of unit of medical time, taking account of both qualitative and quantitative factors. The points awarded should reflect time, intensity of workload, inconvenience and any need for an incentive. Once agreed, they should be entered in the appropriate column along line 7, between charts 1 and 2.

When calculating values in chart 2, it should be noted that scores in chart 1 which relate to weekly workload should be multiplied by 52 to obtain the point score for the equivalent column of chart 2 (eg: $A = (a \times 52) \times$ number of points; $B = (b \times 52) \times$ number of points). The numbers in chart 1 which relate to annual workload patterns should be multiplied by the actual number of points in the same column; the resulting multiple should be then included in the corresponding column of chart 2 (eg $F = f \times$ number of points).

Chart 3 contains the adjustment factor given to each partner according to their position in relation to parity: parity scores 1.0 whereas a new partner on a 60% share scores 0.6. When chart 2 is completed, individual subtotals are calculated for chart 3 by adding together the numbers in each line for each partner (eg, for Dr J, the scores represented by letters A, B, etc, to H should be added together to yield Dr J's individual subtotal). Individual subtotals should be multiplied by the agreed adjustment factors to obtain individual totals. The practice total is obtained by adding together all individual totals. Profit sharing ratios (expressed as percentages) are obtained by dividing the practice total by each individual total, and then multiplying by 100.

Conclusion

This chapter has described a far more formal approach to measuring partners' workload than is found in the large majority of practices. Although it may appear to be too rigid for some practices, it can serve as a benchmark against which to assess more informal ways of measuring workload. A key feature is its capacity to relate in a tabular form the principal factors which should ultimately determine each partner's profit share:

- the amount and type of actual work done
- relative weighting given to different types of work
- the practice's profit sharing ratio.

Irrespective of how formalized, systematic or scientific your method of measuring workload may be, its credibility ultimately depends upon qualitative judgements which underlie practice agreements, in particular key judgements relating to the workload implications of different types of work (eg surgery consultations and night visits, various clinical conditions and various types of consultations).

9 Improving Partnership Agreements

Tony Stanton

THERE is probably no such thing as a perfect partnership agreement. Tempting though the prospect may be, to promulgate a single template, and claim that any practice can use it when drawing up its partnership agreement, would prove a fruitless task. This is because there are such wide variations between practice circumstances and greatly differing personalities and idiosyncrasies among partners, and because NHS general practice itself is continually changing.

When attempting to improve a partnership agreement, it is essential to keep the following key parameters in mind:

- the content of partnership law, in particular the 1890 Partnership Act
- the NHS General Medical Services Regulations 1992
- the NHS Statement of Fees and Allowances (the Red Book).

Arguably the most fundamental question is the one which is probably most rarely asked; namely, what is the overriding purpose of a partnership agreement? It is certainly not a document to which doctors would expect to refer routinely. In essence, it is a framework on which successful working relationships depend and is more concerned with binding people together than enabling the expulsion of partners.

Given the continuing trend towards an increase in both the number and size of partnerships, together with more opportunities to vary individual GPs' hours of availability, we are likely to see more, rather than fewer, occasions when partnership agreements need to be referred to and/or amended. There is a lot to be said for seizing the opportunity of a partner's retirement, the appointment of an additional partner, or an application to change a partner's hours of availability, to review the partnership agreement itself.

Bearing in mind that there is no such thing as an ideal model agreement, it is important to recognize that each individual partnership agreement should reflect the detailed thoughts and decisions of the partners themselves (and/or prospective partners) on how they wish to work together. The job of the partnership's legal advisers is to prepare a clear legal statement of the arrangements the partners wish to make.

Ideally, a new partnership deed should be entered into immediately before a new partner actually joins a partnership. It is certainly sensible that a new partner should be invited to obtain his or her own independent legal advice.

A profound development, which has taken place in NHS general practice over the past generation or so, has been the propensity of partnerships to appoint incoming doctors immediately as partners in their practices. There are two main reasons for this: firstly that doctors admitted as partners normally qualify for the basic practice allowance and its related allowances; and secondly the laudable desire of many practices to avoid, at almost any cost, being guilty of the type of exploitation traditionally associated with the employment of an assistant 'with a view' to becoming a partner – particularly since, in some cases, the view was so distant that it represented a limitless and unreachable horizon. Nevertheless, there is a powerful argument that both the newcomer and the existing partners could be better served by the employment of an assistant 'with a view' for a period of, say, six months, to enable there to be mutual assessment, following which a genuine offer of a partnership could be made, which would lead to parity within a definite and reasonable timescale.

A basic framework for a partnership

The basic framework described below includes a number of essential building blocks which need to be considered when seeking to improve partnership agreements. As with any building, a strong foundation is needed and the inscription on the foundation stone should include a definition of the life expectancy of the partnership. This may be for a fixed period, or for the joint lives of all the partners or any two of them.

The agreement should refer to the effect on the partnership of a voluntary or compulsory retirement of one of its partners. Although NHS GPs are obliged to retire from the FHSA medical list at age 70, a doctor who is 70 or over may serve as a locum or assistant to a principal on an FHSA medical list. Moreover, many practices engage in significant amounts of non-NHS work and thought should therefore be given as to whether a partner who retires from NHS general practice may continue to undertake other work within the partnership. Doctors are looking increasingly towards earlier, rather than later, retirement ages and there is much to be said for including a normal retirement age in the partnership agreement.

A fundamental point to consider, when drawing up the partnership agreement, is the effect of the Sex Discrimination Act 1975, which makes it unlawful to discriminate against a woman who is seeking employment or a partnership, or a woman already working as an employee or partner. It should be noted that discrimination has a fairly broad definition under the provisions of the Act; it includes the application of terms or conditions in an agreement which, although applicable in theory to men and women equally, have a disproportional impact which is disadvantageous to a woman.

It is vital to remember that each partner has to discharge the duties and exercise the powers of a principal in relation to the running of the practice. This fundamental requirement is built into the NHS regulations. If it is not complied with, the FHSA will be able to regard the doctor concerned as an assistant and not a principal.

Availability and profit shares

A further area of potential confusion concerns the relationship in the NHS regulations between approved hours of availability and minimum share of profits.

- A doctor whose approved hours are not less than 26 hours per week is entitled to a share of the profits which is not less than one third of the share of the partner with the greatest share.

- A doctor whose approved hours are less than 26 hours per week, but not less than 19 hours a week, is entitled to a share of the profits not less than one quarter of the share of the partner with the greatest share.

- A doctor whose approved hours are less than 19 hours per week, but not less than 13 hours per week, is entitled to a share of the profits not less than one fifth of the share of the partner with the greatest share.

For the purposes of these requirements, job sharers are regarded as one whole person. The fractions of the profit shares are minimum shares. Profit shares should reflect the actual workload of individual partners, which is quite a separate matter from hours of availability.

As well as specifying the profit sharing arrangement, the agreement should also clearly define the time taken to reach parity and the steps to be taken on the way. The arrangements for profit sharing should also be free from any conditions, such as list size, bearing in mind that the Medical Practices Committee has stated that, if the period taken to reach parity exceeds three years, there may be a hidden sale of goodwill.

Understandably, some doctors will wish to limit the extent of their commitment to the partnership, in terms of hours of availability or duties undertaken, and the partnership agreement will need to provide for an appropriate level of remuneration. The concept of a salaried partner should be avoided. In the case of partners not having a full-time commitment to the practice, special care is needed when calculating their profit share ratios. The requirements of the regulations summarized on page 103 apply to all partners. Very great care needs to be taken if such payments are defined as a fixed sum. It may be safer to define them as a fixed proportion which must be not less than a specified fixed sum, thereby satisfying not only the NHS regulations but the reasonable expectations of the partner concerned. There is a powerful argument that a partner with a guaranteed share of this type should at least have the option of becoming a full profit sharing partner in agreed circumstances, eg if there is a change in the constitution or circumstances of the partnership.

A checklist of key financial issues

There is no doubt that dissatisfaction with financial arrangements is a common cause of partnership disagreements. It is therefore essential that the partnership agreement should be capable of providing clear and unambiguous answers to the following key questions.

- How is practice income defined?
- How are NHS allowances distributed among the partners?
- How is income from outside the NHS distributed among the partners?
- Which expenses are charged to the partnership, and which are paid by partners individually?
- Is the partnership bank account held in the names of all partners or of the practice?
- Are all partners included in the bank mandate?
- Is there an agreed basis of cheque signing?

- Are the practice accountants named in the deed, and does it make provision for each partner to receive the annual accounts and to have access to the practice's bank statements?

As well as addressing these financial issues, the partnership deed should define the capital assets used by the practice and the arrangements for incoming partners to acquire appropriate shares – leading to a parity share – in such assets. The difference between these capital assets and the partnership capital is described in Chapter 5. Partnership capital must also be defined clearly. The deed will need to specify how capital assets are valued, the basis of ownership and how shares in those assets are bought and sold.

Since practice premises are at the very heart of a practice's viability, the deed must specify the basis of the occupation of all premises, whether they are owned, leased or held on a licence. In the case of joint ownership of premises, there needs to be an agreed basis of valuation for all incoming and outgoing interested partners. If the premises have been developed under the cost rent scheme, there is a powerful argument in favour of a specific formula for valuation. It is not uncommon for premises to be owned by an individual partner, in which case there needs to be a clear statement as to whether the value of such interests is included or excluded from the partnership capital. The security of tenure for the partnership and sensible arrangements for disposal of such interests must also be included in the deed.

Leave arrangements

Leave entitlement is another common cause of unhappiness. The basis for leave entitlement for holidays, sickness, study and maternity should be defined clearly. Partners should have an equitable entitlement to holiday and study leave. The deed should include the arrangements for sickness, specifying whether the cost of employing a locum is the responsibility of the individual partners or the partnership as a whole. There should be a clear understanding as to whether the individual or the partnership receives any 'sickness related' income from the FHSA or a sickness insurance policy.

Maternity leave arrangements are a particularly sensitive area. Fourteen weeks absence should be regarded as the minimum length and the partner concerned should be free to choose when to start her maternity leave, in consultation with her own medical advisers. It could well be regarded as discriminatory on grounds of sex if a partnership's maternity leave provisions are less advantageous than those for sick leave. Similarly, if a partner takes maternity leave, she should not lose her entitlement to pro-rata holiday and sickness leave in respect of this period. Not all women wish to return to work after childbirth and the inclusion of a maximum period of absence in the partnership agreement might be a sensible precaution. It may also be advisable to agree arrangements for adoption leave, although as yet there are no hard and fast guidelines in this area.

Professional obligations

The remaining block of issues to be considered when building better partnership agreements relates to the matter of professional obligations. A key difficulty is that there is no such thing as a job description for a GP. However, a statement of the partners' obligations to each other, not only that they should conduct themselves properly in the best interests of the practice, but also that they should take all necessary steps to comply with the requirements of their terms and conditions of service, helps to set an appropriate ethos for the practice. It follows that all patients attending the practice should have the right to register with the partner of their choice, subject only to the agreement of the partner concerned.

As well as making clear provisions for the normal retirement of a partner from the practice, the partnership agreement also needs to include clear provisions relating to the dissolution of the partnership. Common sense also dictates that there should be specific provision for the resolution of disputes.

Fundamental to all these considerations is the need to agree how partnership decisions are to be taken, including reference to the voting position of part-time and job sharing partners. There are a number of levels at which partnership decisions are required: on day to day matters, on matters of policy (which might require the unanimous vote of all partners), and in those circumstances where there is a need to take an urgent decision which does not involve a change of partnership policy. These latter considerations being us back to the point made earlier about the need to define the purpose behind setting up a partnership in the first instance.

Partnerships and personalities

At the end of the day, the partnership agreement is only a legal framework to enable a team of doctors to work together both successfully and (one hopes) happily. Preparing, revising and improving partnership agreements helps to concentrate minds. Sadly, however, many partnership breakdowns are due to far less tangible issues than those capable of being addressed in a partnership agreement. These problems are much more concerned with personality differences, not all of which are either foreseeable or even soluble. Obviously some can be avoided by having a period of mutual assessment of a reasonable duration, as discussed on page 102.

Although the actual work which an individual GP does with patients is intensely personal, the success of a general practice partnership depends on the successful bonding of individuals into a reasonably happy team. This requires a mixture of different skills and personalities. A successful practice is likely to have people prepared to innovate, good organizers, natural conciliators and a mixture of talents. Although all this may seem self-evident, many doctors fail to recognize it.

Partnerships faced with an impending change may think it sensible to invest in psychometric profiling. Such a process draws attention to the personalities and qualities of the existing partners, and may well help to identify a missing piece or pieces in the jigsaw. Profiling shortlisted candidates should help to identify the strengths and weaknesses of individual applicants, and improve the chance of recruiting the person most suited to becoming a good team member. Although this can be a comparatively expensive exercise, it may prove to be a very worthwhile investment.

10 Future Developments

Simon Fradd

ALTHOUGH the way in which general practice delivers its services has changed dramatically over the last decade, its legal framework has barely altered since the inception of the NHS. Independent contractor status has prevailed in all but a few exceptional circumstances. A large majority of GPs continue to work as either single-handed doctors or in partnerships, not as employees. Any changes to this basic framework have been so marginal that they are barely discernible. Even the Government's controversial fundholding initiative has challenged neither GPs' independent contractor status nor their partnership arrangements. Fundholding may have increased the strain of working in a partnership, but it has not in itself affected the basic concept.

It is perhaps significant that, in the few cases where doctors have been 'employed' to provide general medical services, the failure rate of such initiatives has been relatively high. It would seem that primary care requires delivery of a flexible and personalized service and that the self-employed status of GPs is ideally suited to ensure that this can be achieved, thereby satisfying the needs and aspirations of both the public and the profession. In particular, it has allowed practices to adapt easily and rapidly to local circumstances, to a far greater extent than larger organizations could ever be capable of achieving.

However, the fact that the legal framework of partnerships has not changed does not mean there have not been any new developments or experiments. Nor does it mean that a single model can or should prevail.

The current legal framework

Traditionally, general practice has been provided by either a single-handed doctor or a partnership of doctors. Non-medical members of the practice team are almost invariably employees of a doctor or the partnership. It used to be normal for there to be a 'hierarchy' among the partners based on seniority, but this arrangement is increasingly being challenged. The NHS income of the partnership (and usually other, non-NHS income as well) generates the practice's profits, and these are shared according to a profit sharing formula agreed between the partners. In some practices one or more partners have a guaranteed minimum share and may be inappropriately termed 'salaried partners'.

NHS regulations impose a legal restriction on the ratios of these profit shares; the lowest earning partner cannot earn less than one third of the profits of the highest earning partner, if both are full-time (this is apportioned proportionally for part-time working, see page 103). Several related influences have led to this restriction on the size of partnership shares, including successive governments' opposition to the sale of goodwill and their wish to ensure that NHS general practice is provided by independent self-employed clinicians, who are partners in their practices and not salaried assistants with or without a view to succession.

The need for change

The primary care team

The 1990 contract, the development of the purchaser-provider model and recent community care legislation have all had a radical impact on how primary care is being delivered. Indeed, prior to the 1980s, it was normal to refer simply to general practice rather than primary care. GPs themselves were responsible for delivering virtually all of their patients' medical care, sometimes assisted by district nurses, midwives and health visitors and (more recently) treatment room/practice nurses. The rest of the team consisted of a receptionist and/or secretary, often part-time. Remarkably, this style of general practice was prevalent until comparatively recently.

GPs worked in partnerships for their own convenience: they allowed cross cover for days off, leave periods and out-of-hours work, and they enabled economies of scale to be achieved through the sharing of receptionists, secretaries and nurses. It was not surprising that the partnerships themselves included only GP principals: they did the clinical work, decided how the practice should be run, took the responsibility and retained the profits.

The development of the primary care team will be a major influence on the future of general practice. Although GPs continue to work in partnerships or as single-handed doctors (albeit often in informal association with one another), they are devolving to their staff an ever increasing proportion of their clinical, management and administrative work. On the one hand, the clinical work of GPs is becoming more specialized in certain respects; for example, as a result of taking on much of the disease management function which was previously in the province of consultants in the hospital sector. GPs are also assuming increased management responsibilities − managing larger teams of staff and budgets; and they are taking on responsibility for commissioning secondary care from the hospital sector. On the other hand, they are devolving much of their routine clinical work to practice nurses, midwives, health visitors, social workers and other health professionals.

GPs can no longer seriously claim to carry sole responsibility for providing primary care. Some would take the argument further by pointing out that GPs cannot even presume to be the obvious leaders of the primary care team. The challenge to their traditional leadership role is coming from several directions. Practice managers not only do the book-keeping; they also hire, fire and train staff. They have special expertise which many doctors lack, such as knowledge of employment law and personnel management. Practice nurses are becoming nurse practitioners, acquiring their own specialist skills. Midwives are anticipating that their profession too could acquire a more autonomous role, if current proposals to change the delivery of midwifery services are implemented. Thus there is no shortage of potential challengers to the GP's leadership role.

Extending the partnership

The reason general practice partnerships consist only of GP principals is due in part to custom and practice. There appears to be no statutory restriction as such on doctors entering into partnership with nurses and others who work in general practice.

Traditionally, general practice comprised a doctor seeing and treating patients, with a receptionist or secretary undertaking clerical and administrative duties. As primary care has developed, more team members have become involved in clinical work, including health visitors, practice nurses and midwives. Alongside these developments, the vast increase in administration has led GPs to delegate more non-clinical work to receptionists, secretaries and practice managers.

At first sight it might appear logical for membership of partnerships to be extended to encompass some of the key staff, notably practice managers and practice nurses. To understand why this has rarely happened, we need to spell out why GPs have opted to work in partnerships.

The reason why two or more doctors, solicitors, accountants and other professionals form a partnership to ply their trade is to share responsibility, risks and expenses, and to obtain financial advantage from economies of scale. They do not opt to work in a partnership simply because this somehow leads to larger financial rewards. Indeed, there is no prima facie evidence to show that GP partners necessarily earn more than their salaried counterparts. Nor does a partnership imply equality of earnings: it is possible for the profit sharing ratio between two GP partners' earnings to be as great as 3:1 under the current regulations.

A major downside of a partnership is that partners are self-employed and do not therefore benefit from the protection of employment legislation, such as that relating to unfair dismissal, sick leave, maternity and unemployment benefits. Partners also carry enormous responsibility for each other's actions and omissions; for example, they are jointly and severally liable for each other's taxation. Above all, one must stress that, by their very nature, working relationships within partnerships are rarely simple or easy. Experience suggests that partners have to make far greater efforts to develop and maintain good working relations than comparable professionals working as colleague employees.

Entering a partnership is also a long-term commitment. At the time of joining, the expectation is generally to continue in the partnership throughout one's working life. Some earnings will not be taken as income, but left instead in the practice to provide working capital. This capital cannot be withdrawn until retirement or dissolution of the partnership. In this way, drawings are reduced throughout a partner's working lifetime.

Sale of goodwill

The sale of goodwill was banned at the inception of the NHS. Traditionally, the money generated by doctors selling their goodwill provided them with funds for their retirement. However, the NHS introduced a special superannuation scheme for GPs, thereby ending the profession's traditional dependence on the lump sum obtained from selling the practice's goodwill. At the time of its abolition, it was widely assumed that the buying and selling of goodwill was contrary to the interests of patients. For example, although a large list size would enhance the value of a doctor's goodwill, having to care for a large number of patients was not generally in their best interests.

The GMSC has just restated its commitment to maintaining the status quo on the issue of goodwill. However, the present position is not without its anomalies. The most obvious of these concerns the value of practice premises, particularly those which are eligible for cost rent reimbursement. Since property values have declined dramatically during the past few years (unprecedented during the period since 1948), some doctors nearing retirement have found that their premises are now worth less than what they paid for them. Nevertheless, current NHS legislation requires practice premises (including partners' shares in them) to be sold at a current valuation, regardless of how much money, time or energy has been invested in them, or how much cost rent income is paid by the FHSA.

It could be argued that the position in relation to cost rent reimbursement is somewhat different. Apart from a single-handed GP, cost rent will continue to be paid to the practice, regardless of any change in membership of the partnership, until and unless the practice opts to change from a cost rent to a notional rent. Thus the income (in the form of direct reimbursements) generated by the premises relates to actual building costs, not their current value. It could be argued that a transfer of ownership of a cost rented surgery at the cost rent value should not constitute a sale of goodwill.

A final note of caution: practices should be very wary of changing from a cost rent to a notional rent. Notional rent can go down as well as up. Recently cases of 40% reduction in notional rent have occurred in some areas.

Personal lists

Some partnerships seem to change their partners almost as frequently as the GP contract is amended! When one investigates these cases, there is often a significant and persistent disparity in personal list sizes between individual partners.

There should be no doubt that patient numbers are power. If one partner has 3500 registered patients and the other only 35, it is not difficult to guess who is likely to fare worse if a dissolution should occur. The profession should address this issue without delay; it should either review the system used by the practice for registering patients, or apply some measure of compulsion which ensures that incoming partners are able to register new patients. Of course senior partners have to be protected from rogue newcomers, but if the former succeed to the original list of a retiring partner, there cannot be too much harm in letting new patients register with the new partner after a short period of mutual assessment.

Index

accounting records 49
accounts 23–4
  accruals basis 44
  direct reimbursements in 49
  and fundholding 55, 58–60
  income and expenditure 43–6
  presentation 46–9
arbitration 24–5, 31
assets 50, 105

balance sheet 49–52
banking arrangements 23
brass plate restriction 88–9
Business Names Act 1985 11

capital, partnership 13, 105
capital accounts 53
capital allowances 63–5, 78
capital grants 46
cars, capital allowances on 63–4
communication 27, 35–7
cost rent 113
court action 30–1, 40
current accounts 53–4
current assets 50
current liabilities 52

debtors 44, 52
defence body subscriptions 22
depreciation 44–5
direct reimbursement 49
discrimination 16, 20, 87–8, 103
disputes, avoiding 27–8
drugs, valuation 44

expenses, partnership 13–14
exploitation in partnerships 81–92

fixed assets 50
forward planning 27–8
fundholding
  bank account 58
  and partnership accounts 55, 58–60
funds, partners 52–5, 56, 57
future developments 109–13

General Medical Services Regulations 1992 82, 83

general practice contract (1990) 4
goodwill 3, 90–1
  protection of 22
  sale of 15–16, 112–13
grossing-up principle 43–4

hearsay 28
holiday entitlement 19, 105
hours of availability and profits 103–4

income, partnership 14
Income and Corporation Taxes Act 1988 39
income tax
  arrangements for 18–19
  assessable profit allocation 65
  basis of assessment 66–8
  calculating liability 66
  calculating profits 63
  capital allowances 63–5
  at cessation of partnership 69
  joint and several liability 66
  in new partnerships 68–9
  overlap relief 77–8
  personal expenses claims 65
  proposed changes for the self-employed 70–9
  provision for 55, 56, 57
injunction 30
interim order 30

job sharers 103

Landlord and Tenant Act 1954 39
lawyers 31, 33
leave advances 53
leave arrangements 20, 105–6
liabilities 52
list size 113
litigation 30–1, 40
locum expenses 20
long-term liabilities 52

management allowance, fundholding 58, 59
mandatory injunction 30
maternity leave 20–1, 105–6
mediation 40–1

Medical Practices Committee (MPC) 3
  and goodwill 15–16, 90–1
  and restrictive covenants 23
  meetings 35–6
  minutes 27–8, 36
  problem-solving 28–9
MPC see Medical Practices Committee

nature of the business 11
NHS General Medical Services
    Regulations 1992 82, 83
non-solicitation clause 89
notice period 21
notional rent 113

open areas 3
out-of-hours commitment 95

parity 94
partners
  display of names 11
  funds 52–5, 56, 57
  legal rights and responsibilities 29–30
  personal expenses 60–1
  property owning 12
  salaried 85–6, 110
partnership
  advantages 1–5
  breakdown 32–3, 37–40
  criteria for 82–7
  decisions by 18
  definition 82
  dissolution 11, 12, 37–41
  duration of 11–12
  exploitation in 81–92
  expulsion from 21
  extension to primary care team
    members 111–12
  genuine 81–2
  joint lives 12, 37
  leaving 21
  maintaining 35–7
  name of 11
  and personality 106–7
Partnership Act 1890 4, 7, 29–30
  and determination of existence of
    partnership 83
  and dissolution of partnerships 12, 37–9
  and partnership decisions 18
partnership agreement
  commencement date 10
  framework 9–25, 102–6
  improving 101–7
  written 7–9

partnership at will 7, 8, 29–30
  dissolution 37–41
penalty clauses 87
personal expenses 60–1, 65, 78
personal lists 113
personality and partnership 106–7
practice area map 22
practice premises
  address 11
  in partnership agreement 11–12, 105
  valuation 12
practice staff
  management of 17–18
  reimbursement in fundholding
    practices 58, 60
pregnancy rights 20, 105–6
primary care team 110–11
  meetings 36
  as members of partnership 111–12
problem-solving 28–9
professional obligations 106
profits
  allocation 14–15, 45–6, 65, 103–4, 110
  calculation 63
  and hours of availability 103–4
  and workload 93–9
property capital accounts 52–3
property owners 12
psychometric profiling 107

restrictive covenants 3, 22, 23, 88–90
retirement 21–2, 102–3

salaried partners 85–6, 110
senior partner 28
sex discrimination 20, 87–8, 103
Sex Discrimination Act 1986 20, 103
SFA see Statement of Fees and Allowances
sickness leave 20, 105
single-handed practice, setting up 3
Statement of Fees and Allowances
    (SFA) 4, 43–4
study leave 19, 105

taxation see income tax
time devoted to practice 16–17

workload
  measurement 93–4
  and profits 93–9
writs 30–1